THIRD EDITION

Documentation Manual for Occupational Therapy
Writing SOAP Notes

THIRD EDITION

Documentation Manual for Occupational Therapy
Writing SOAP Notes

CRYSTAL A. GATELEY, MA, OTR/L
CLINICAL ASSISTANT PROFESSOR
UNIVERSITY OF MISSOURI
COLUMBIA, MISSOURI

SHERRY BORCHERDING, MA, OTR/L
CLINICAL ASSOCIATE PROFESSOR, RETIRED
UNIVERSITY OF MISSOURI
COLUMBIA, MISSOURI

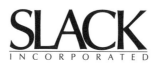

SLACK
INCORPORATED

www.slackbooks.com

ISBN: 978-1-55642-971-2

Copyright © 2012 by SLACK Incorporated

Instructors: Documentation Manual for Occupational Therapy: Writing SOAP Notes, Third Edition Instructor's Manual is also available from SLACK Incorporated. Don't miss this important companion to *Documentation Manual for Occupational Therapy: Writing SOAP Notes, Third Edition.* To obtain the Instructor's Manual, please visit http://www.efacultylounge.com.

Crystal A. Gateley and *Sherry Borcherding* have no financial or proprietary interest in the materials presented herein.

The procedures and practices described in this book should be implemented in a manner consistent with the professional standards set for the circumstances that apply in each specific situation. Every effort has been made to confirm the accuracy of the information presented and to correctly relate generally accepted practices. The authors, editor, and publisher cannot accept responsibility for errors or exclusions or for the outcome of the material presented herein. There is no expressed or implied warranty of this book or information imparted by it. Any review or mention of specific companies or products is not intended as an endorsement by the author or publisher.

SLACK Incorporated uses a review process to evaluate submitted material. Prior to publication, educators or clinicians provide important feedback on the content that we publish. We welcome feedback on this work.

Published by: SLACK Incorporated
6900 Grove Road
Thorofare, NJ 08086 USA
Telephone: 856-848-1000
Fax: 856-853-5991
www.slackbooks.com

Contact SLACK Incorporated for more information about other books in this field or about the availability of our books from distributors outside the United States.

Library of Congress Cataloging-in-Publication Data

Gateley, Crystal A., 1974-
    Documentation manual for occupational therapy : writing SOAP notes / Crystal A. Gateley, Sherry Borcherding. -- 3rd ed.
        p. ; cm.
    Rev. ed. of: Documentation manual for writing SOAP notes in occupational therapy / Sherry Borcherding. 2nd ed. c2005.
    Includes bibliographical references and index.
    ISBN 978-1-55642-971-2 (alk. paper)
    1. Occupational therapy--Documentation--Handbooks, manuals, etc. 2. Medical protocols--Handbooks, manuals, etc. 3. Medical records--Handbooks, manuals, etc. I. Borcherding, Sherry. II. Borcherding, Sherry. Documentation manual for writing SOAP notes in occupational therapy. III. Title.
    [DNLM: 1. Forms and Records Control--Handbooks. 2. Occupational Therapy--methods--Handbooks. 3. Medical Records--Handbooks. 4. Patient Care Planning--Handbooks. 5. Writing--Handbooks. WB 39]
    RM735.4.B67 2011
    615.8'515--dc23
                                        2011012981

Last digit is print number: 10   9   8   7   6   5

DEDICATION

This book is dedicated to all of my past, current, and future OT students who make teaching a wonderful and rewarding experience. It is my hope that this book will serve you in your endeavors to provide compassionate care to your clients and to communicate the benefit of the occupational therapy profession.

Crystal A. Gateley, MA, OTR/L

This book is dedicated to the occupational therapy students, faculty, and fieldwork instructors who have taught me so much about documentation, and to my grandson, Jan, who carries on the family tradition in occupational therapy.

Sherry Borcherding, MA, OTR/L

CONTENTS

Instructors: *Documentation Manual for Occupational Therapy: Writing SOAP Notes, Third Edition Instructor's Manual* is also available from SLACK Incorporated. Don't miss this important companion to *Documentation Manual for Occupational Therapy: Writing SOAP Notes, Third Edition*. To obtain the Instructor's Manual, please visit http://www.efacultylounge.com.

ACKNOWLEDGMENTS

I would like to thank Sherry Borcherding for teaching me how to document long ago as a student, for her support and encouragement over the past two decades, and for her trust in me to serve as coauthor on this project. I would also like to thank Brien Cummings and the staff at SLACK Incorporated who tolerated my never-ending questions throughout the revision process.

I am grateful to Diana Baldwin who has been the impetus for my educational and professional advancement on multiple occasions, and to Guy McCormack and Diane Smith for their support as I worked on this project. I would like to thank Leanna Garrison, Molly Tugushi, and M. Boden Lyon for their patience and assistance with my technology questions.

I am grateful to my long-time friend Jeffrey Sable for his encouragement from afar and for the humorous emails that kept me smiling on days when I thought I might never finish this project. I also appreciate the support of my Wakonse Fellows, whose friendship and humor make my days enjoyable.

A big thank you goes out to the many University of Missouri OT students who have allowed their notes to be used in this book to teach others. I especially want to thank the Classes of 2011 and 2012 who provided considerable feedback and editing during the revision process. I would also like to acknowledge the contributions of Vic Zuccarello, David McSpadden, Shelia Tenny, Joe Sadewhite, Patty Daus, Kathy Nelson, Stephanie Schmidt, Shawna Dunnaway, Michelle Wheeler, Kayla Harmon, and Melanie Cook in helping us make certain that the content of this book is consistent with current occupational therapy practice.

Most importantly, I would like to thank my husband, Curt, and my two daughters, Katrina and Lauren, whose patience, love, and support continue to be my inspiration in life.

Crystal A. Gateley, MA, OTR/L

Many people have contributed to the development of this manual. First I would like to thank Crystal Gateley for joining me as coauthor on this 3rd edition. Her upgrades to the manual have taken it to another level. I would like to thank Diana Baldwin for her patience in teaching me how to teach. Without her nurturing and support, I might have taken another pathway entirely. Thanks to Fred Dittrich for moving me as gracefully and quickly into the Information Age as I could tolerate. Thanks to Sandy Matsuda for her editing contributions, and for her loving friendship and support. Thanks to Doris O'Hara for bequeathing me the basic course material many years ago, and to Charlet Quay, Stephanie Owings, David Lackey, Lynne White, Lea Ann Lowery, and Carol Kappel for filling in the gaps in my knowledge base. Thanks to Leanna Garrison for being the Format Goddess. Thanks to Theresa Lackey, Chris Nelson, Linda Eagle and Randy Kilgore for their help and support. But most of all, I would like to thank the occupational therapy classes at the University of Missouri, who allowed their notes to be used to teach others.

Sherry Borcherding, MA, OTR/L

ABOUT THE AUTHORS

Crystal A. Gateley, MA, OTR/L currently serves as a faculty member at University of Missouri in Columbia where she has taught since 2009. She teaches Foundations of Occupation, Developmental Framework, Pediatric Fieldwork, Clinical Documentation, and Health & Wellness. She has also taught Advanced Strategies and Problem-Based Cases. Crystal also assists with supervising occupational therapy students at the program's on-site pediatric clinic.

Crystal graduated Summa Cum Laude from University of Missouri with a BHS in occupational therapy and went on to complete her master's in educational leadership and policy analysis (ELPA), also from the University of Missouri. She is currently pursuing a doctoral degree in ELPA from the University of Missouri. Crystal has worked in a variety of OT practice settings, including inpatient and outpatient rehabilitation, long-term care, home health, outpatient pediatrics, public schools, and sheltered workshops.

Besides teaching, Crystal enjoys attending her daughters' extracurricular events, including soccer, basketball, and band. She also loves camping, fishing, and boating with family and friends.

Sherry Borcherding, MA, OTR/L recently retired from the faculty of University of Missouri where she taught for 15 years. During the time she was on faculty, she taught disability awareness; complementary therapy; clinical ethics; frames of reference; psychopathology; loss and disability; long-term care; wellness; and a three-semester fieldwork sequence designed to develop critical thinking, clinical reasoning, and documentation skills. Two of her courses were designated as campus writing courses and one was credentialed for computer and information proficiency. As a part of the fieldwork and documentation courses, she filmed simulated occupational therapy interventions for student use in class. Three of those "movies" are available on www.efacultylounge.com with this edition of the book.

Sherry graduated with honors from Texas Woman's University, Denton with a BS in occupational therapy and went on to complete her master's in special education with special faculty commendation at George Peabody College, Nashville, Tennessee. Following her staff positions in rehabilitation, home health, and pediatrics, she assumed a number of management roles including Chief Occupational Therapist at East Texas Treatment Center, Kilgore; Director of Occupational Therapy at Mid-Missouri Mental Health Center, Columbia; and Director of Rehabilitation Services at Transitional Housing Agency, Columbia, Missouri. She has also planned, designed and directed occupational therapy programs at Capital Regional Medical Center, Jefferson City, Missouri and at Charter Behavioral Health Center, Columbia, Missouri.

Sherry is a lifelong learner. Since her retirement, she has further expanded her private practice devoted to complementary and alternative therapies. She is certified in CranioSacral Therapy at the techniques level through Upledger Institute, Palm Beach Gardens, Florida and is attuned as a Reiki master. For leisure, Sherry enjoys music, dance, and all kinds of three-dimensional art. Her pottery has appeared in several local shows over the past few years.

Documenting the Occupational Therapy Process

Welcome to a new style of writing. The first time you see an experienced occupational therapist make an entry in a health record, you may be tempted to think you will never be able to do it. The technical language alone can be intimidating. Then there is the amazing attention to detail in the client observation, the insightful assessment, and the plan that just seems to roll off the therapist's fingertips while you are wondering how long it will take you to be able to predict a course of treatment like that.

Professional documentation is a skill, and like any skill, it can be learned. Learning a new skill requires two things: instruction and practice. This manual is designed to provide you with both parts of the process. Information is presented on each part of the documentation process, and the worksheets are designed to let you practice each step as you learn it.

The material presented here grew out of a course on clinical documentation taught to senior occupational therapy students at the University of Missouri. It has been field-tested to be sure it is understandable and effective in helping you learn both documentation and clinical-reasoning skills.

Occupational therapy practitioners write in many different formats depending on their practice settings. The purpose of this manual is to present a systematic approach to one form of documentation: the SOAP note. SOAP is an acronym for the four parts of an entry into a health record. The letters stand for *Subjective, Objective, Assessment,* and *Plan.* These terms and their origins are further explained in Chapter 2. The format taught in this manual is one that is reimbursable by most third-party payers, including Medicare. If you learn to meet these standards consistently, you are unlikely to be denied reimbursement for your services. The skills learned through the use of the SOAP note format can be adapted to fit the documentation requirements of nearly any occupational therapy practice setting, including those that use an electronic documentation system.

OUR EVOLVING PROFESSION

The content of this manual is reflective of contemporary occupational therapy practice. As the American Occupational Therapy Association (AOTA) approaches its 100th anniversary in 2017, the following statement has been adopted as the Centennial Vision for the profession:

> We envision that occupational therapy is a powerful, widely recognized, science-driven and evidence-based profession with a globally connected and diverse workforce meeting society's occupational needs (AOTA, 2006a).

This vision statement is intended to serve as a roadmap for all aspects of professional practice, including documentation. Current occupational therapy practice is in many ways determined by which services are reimbursable, and documentation of client care is the vehicle by which those services are communicated. As the profession continues the move toward evidence-based practice, well-documented occupational therapy services are more likely to be recognized and reimbursed as a cost-effective treatment in improving health and quality of life (Clark & Bloom, 2006).

Gateley CA, Borcherding S. *Documentation Manual for Occupational Therapy: Writing SOAP Notes, 3rd Edition* (pp. 1-6)
© 2012 SLACK Incorporated

Occupational therapists are challenged with combining the ever-changing knowledge base of the profession with its historical foundations and this visionary roadmap for the future. Crepeau, Boyt Schell, and Cohn (2009a) identified three principles to guide contemporary occupational therapy:

1. Client-centered practice
2. Occupation-centered practice
3. Evidence-based practice

Clinical documentation in occupational therapy must reflect these principles. Occupational therapists must collaborate with clients during evaluation and intervention to ensure that clients have an active role in their care, and that collaboration should be documented throughout the therapeutic process. The targeted outcome of occupational therapy intervention is enhanced engagement in meaningful occupations, and the documented goals and interventions should have occupation as a central theme. Finally, occupational therapists should be documenting assessments and interventions that represent the best evidence available for addressing a client's specific needs.

OUR EVOLVING PROFESSIONAL LANGUAGE

INTERNATIONAL CLASSIFICATION OF FUNCTIONING, DISABILITY AND HEALTH

The *International Classification of Functioning, Disability and Health* (World Health Organization [WHO], 2001), known commonly as ICF, was published by WHO to provide a common language and framework for describing health and disability. The ICF is based on a biopsychosocial model that views disability and function as the "outcomes of interactions between health conditions…and contextual factors" (WHO, 2002, p. 9). Health conditions include diseases, disorders, and injuries. Contextual factors include personal factors as well as environmental factors. In this model (Figure 1-1), function is classified at three levels:

1. Body functions and structure
2. Individual activity
3. Participation in society

Figure 1-1. ICF model of disability. (Reprinted with permission from World Health Organization. (2002). *Towards a common language for functioning, disability and health: ICF.* Geneva, Switzerland: Author. Retrieved from http://www.who.int/classifications/icf/training/icfbeginnersguide.pdf.)

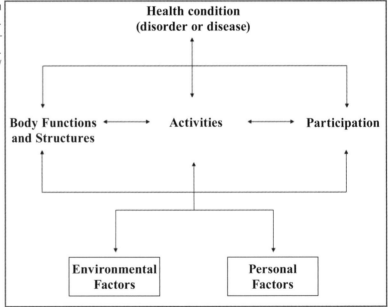

The ICF has been described as "the universal translator," meaning that its standard language can be used for communication across countries, disciplines, and populations (Brachtesende, 2005, p. 14). The concepts presented in the ICF are useful to many health professionals, including occupational therapists, in communicating with team members of other disciplines and with external parties, such as funding sources. In addition, the ICF provides a framework and vocabulary useful to occupational therapists in the documentation of assessments, goals, interventions, and outcomes (Darzins, Fone, & Darzins, 2006).

OCCUPATIONAL THERAPY PRACTICE FRAMEWORK: DOMAIN & PROCESS, 2ND EDITION

While the ICF is a useful tool for occupational therapists in thinking about health and disability, that classification system alone is not sufficient as the language of the profession (Haglund & Henriksson, 2003; Hemmingsson & Jonsson, 2005). More than three decades ago, leaders in the profession recognized the need for a system of uniform terminology. The original document, *Occupational Therapy Product Output Reporting System and Uniform Terminology for Reporting Occupational Therapy Services*, was developed in response to a change in public laws targeted at reducing fraud and abuse of the Medicare and Medicaid systems (AOTA, 1989).

That original document has been revised multiple times and ultimately resulted in the development of the *Occupational Therapy Practice Framework: Domain & Process, 2nd Edition* (*Framework-II*; AOTA, 2008b). The *Framework-II* is the document that defines and guides the professional practice of occupational therapists and occupational therapy assistants. More specifically, the *Framework-II* "was developed to articulate occupational therapy's contribution to promoting the health and participation of people, organizations, and populations through engagement in occupation" (AOTA, 2008b, p. 625). The *Framework-II* is divided into two key sections:

1. *Domain*: This section of the document outlines the scope of occupational therapy and identifies the areas in which occupational therapy practitioners have knowledge and expertise.

2. *Process*: This section focuses on the delivery of occupational therapy services, with a focus on occupation-centered and client-centered practices.

The aspects of occupational therapy's domain (Figure 1-2) are viewed as having a transactional relationship, meaning the various aspects continually influence one another through a reciprocal ongoing relationship (AOTA, 2008b; Dickie, Cutchin, & Humphry, 2006). While the ultimate goal of occupational therapy is to support a client's engagement in meaningful occupation, note that the figure does not imply a hierarchy. The expertise of an occupational therapy practitioner is required to understand and document the relationship between all aspects and the resulting impact on a client's engagement in areas of occupation.

AREAS OF OCCUPATION	CLIENT FACTORS	PERFORMANCE SKILLS	PERFORMANCE PATTERNS	CONTEXT AND ENVIRONMENT	ACTIVITY DEMANDS
Activities of daily living (ADLs)*	Values, beliefs, and spirituality	Sensory perceptual skills	Habits	Cultural	Objects used and their properties
Instrumental activities of daily living (IADLs)	Body functions	Motor and praxis skills	Routines	Personal	Space demands
Rest and sleep	Body structures		Roles	Physical	Social demands
Education		Emotional regulation skills	Rituals	Social	Sequencing and timing
Work		Cognitive skills		Temporal	Required actions
Play		Communication and social skills		Virtual	Required body functions
Leisure					Required body structures
Social participation					
*Also referred to as basic activities of daily living (BADLs) or personal activities of daily living (PADLs)					

Figure 1-2. Domain of occupational therapy. (Reprinted with permission from American Occupational Therapy Association. (2008). Occupational therapy practice framework: Domain & process, 2nd edition. *The American Journal of Occupational Therapy, 62*(6), 625-688.)

The process of service delivery in occupational therapy (Figure 1-3) is composed of evaluation, intervention, and monitoring of outcomes. The *Framework-II* explains that the process of service delivery does not occur in a linear fashion. It is a dynamic process that allows occupational therapy practitioners to continually assess and address a client's needs while focusing on the intended outcome of "supporting health and participation in life through engagement in occupation" (AOTA, 2008b, p. 660). Accurate and effective clinical documentation during all phases of service delivery is essential to communicate the necessity and benefit of occupational therapy to all involved parties.

Diamant (2004) suggests that occupational therapy practitioners could integrate the concepts from the ICF and the *Framework-II* and apply them in practice. The ICF concepts of activities and participation are in alignment with documenting a client's occupational profile during the evaluation process. The concepts of context

---

EVALUATION

Occupational Profile—The initial step in the evaluation process that provides an understanding of the client's occupational history and experiences, patterns of daily living, interests, values, and needs. The client's problems and concerns about performing occupations and daily life activities are identified, and the client's priorities are determined.

Analysis of occupational performance—The step in the evaluation process during which the client's assets, problems, or potential problems are more specifically identified. Actual performance is often observed in context to identify what supports performance and what hinders performance. Performance skills, performance patterns, context or contexts, activity demands, and client factors are all considered, but only selected aspects may be specifically assessed. Targeted outcomes are identified.

INTERVENTION

Intervention plan—A plan that will guide actions taken and that is developed in collaboration with the client. It is based on selected theories, frames of reference, and evidence. Outcomes to be targeted are confirmed.

Intervention implementation—Ongoing actions taken to influence and support improved client performance. Interventions are directed at identified outcomes. Client's response is monitored and documented.

Intervention review—A review of the implementation plan and process as well as its progress toward targeted outcomes.

OUTCOMES (SUPPORTING HEALTH AND PARTICIPATION IN LIFE THROUGH ENGAGEMENT IN OCCUPATION)

Outcomes—Determination of success in reaching designed targeted outcomes. Outcome assessment information is used to plan future actions with the client and to evaluate the service program (i.e., program evaluation).

Figure 1-3. Process of occupational therapy service delivery. (Reprinted with permission from American Occupational Therapy Association. (2008). Occupational therapy practice framework: Domain & process, 2nd edition. *The American Journal of Occupational Therapy, 62*(6), 625-688.)

from the *Framework-II* and contextual factors from the ICF impact a client's participation in areas of occupation, and that impact should be included when documenting evaluation, intervention, and outcomes. Finally, multiple concepts from both documents can be applied in planning and documenting occupation-based and client-centered interventions for clients.

OTHER PUBLICATIONS OF THE AMERICAN OCCUPATIONAL THERAPY ASSOCIATION

The content of this manual reflects the domain and process of contemporary occupational therapy practice as described in the *Framework-II*. AOTA has also published *The Guide to Occupational Therapy Practice, 2nd Edition* (Moyers & Dale, 2007), which reviews the domain and process of the profession and further explains the critical reasoning and decision-making process that occupational therapy practitioners must use in all steps of service delivery. In addition, AOTA publishes numerous *Official Documents* that serve to clarify fundamental concepts of the profession, convey official stances of the profession on relevant issues, and guide education and practice by describing specific principles and procedures in the profession of occupational therapy (Hartmann, 2008). This manual incorporates concepts and guidelines found in the following *Official Documents* of the AOTA:

+ *Scope of Practice* (AOTA, 2010c)
+ *Standards of Practice for Occupational Therapy* (AOTA, 2010d)
+ *Guidelines for Documentation of Occupational Therapy* (AOTA, 2008a)
+ *Guidelines for Supervision, Roles, and Responsibilities During the Delivery of Occupational Therapy Services* (AOTA, 2009)
+ *Occupational Therapy Code of Ethics and Ethics Standards* (AOTA, 2010a)

The Accreditation Council for Occupational Therapy Education (ACOTE) of the AOTA publishes accreditation standards for educational programs at the levels of occupational therapy assistant, master's degree, and doctoral degree. This manual will provide you with a tool for becoming competent in the documentation skills specified in the accreditation standards. While many standards vary according to the requirements of each educational level, the standards for documentation are consistent across all three levels:

+ Standard B.4.10 for the doctoral and master's levels and Standard B.4.6 for the assistant level state that the student will "document occupational therapy services to ensure accountability of service provision and to meet standards for reimbursement of services, adhering to applicable facility, local, state, federal, and reimbursement agencies. Documentation must effectively communicate the need and rationale for occupational therapy services" (AOTA, 2007a, p. 646; 2007b, p. 657; 2007c, p. 667).
+ Standard B.5.28 for the doctoral and master's levels and Standard B.5.27 for the assistant level further stipulates that documentation "must be appropriate to the context in which the service is delivered" (AOTA, 2007a, p. 648; 2007b, p. 658; 2007c, p. 668)

In summary, there are numerous documents and publications that impact the occupational therapy profession as a whole and clinical documentation in particular. It is the responsibility of each occupational therapy practitioner to be familiar with current literature, standards, and state and federal regulations that impact documentation. Leaders in the profession are continually researching and publishing both revised and novel works that impact occupational therapy practice. Additionally, each *Official Document* of the AOTA is reviewed at least every 5 years and revised as needed to reflect current education and practice (Hartmann, 2008). Staying current with all professional publications allows occupational therapy practitioners to engage in evidence-based practice, and this must be reflected in their clinical documentation.

OVERVIEW

The information in this manual has been arranged in the order that it is most easily learned, with foundational concepts presented first. More complex concepts build on these as clinical reasoning is developed. Chapter 2: The Health Record provides an introduction to the medical (health) record, including its function, uses, and history. Chapter 3: Reimbursement, Legal, and Ethical Considerations expands on some of the issues introduced in the previous chapter and provides a general foundation of information to guide documentation in occupational therapy practices. Chapter 4: General Guidelines for Documentation presents the rules and mechanics of documentation.

Chapter 5: Writing Functional Problem Statements discusses the process of developing functional problem statements that can be positively impacted by occupational therapy intervention. Chapter 6: Writing Measurable Occupation-Based Goals and Objectives introduces a new format (COAST) for writing goals and objectives. Worksheets are provided for practice and several examples of problems and goal statements are provided for your reference.

Chapters 7 through 10 teach the four sections of the SOAP format (Subjective, Objective, Assessment, and Plan), which are introduced and explained in Chapters 1 and 2. Multiple examples are presented for each section, and worksheets are provided for practice. Chapter 11: Making Good Notes Even Better reviews the skills presented in the previous six chapters and provides multiple worksheets to refine those skills. Chapter 12: Intervention Planning introduces the intervention planning process that follows an evaluation and provides worksheets to practice this skill.

The last three chapters of this manual serve as a reference as you learn how to document occupational therapy practice. Chapter 13: Documenting Different Stages of Service Delivery presents information from *Guidelines for Documentation of Occupational Therapy* (AOTA, 2008a) and provides examples of documentation from the different stages of the occupational therapy process. Chapter 14: Documentation in Different Practice Settings discusses requirements specific to various settings and funding sources and provides several examples. Chapter 15: Examples of Different Kinds of Notes provides an array of examples from various stages of the occupational therapy process and numerous practice settings.

An appendix with suggestions for completing the worksheets is also provided. It is important to remember that there are multiple "correct" ways to document. As you work through this manual, we recommend that you complete the worksheets on your own **before** looking at the suggested answers in the appendix.

NEW IN THIS EDITION

The third edition of *Documentation Manual for Occupational Therapy: Writing SOAP Notes* is based on the *Occupational Therapy Practice Framework: Domain & Process, 2nd Edition* (AOTA, 2008b) and on the *Guidelines for Documentation of Occupational Therapy* (AOTA, 2008a). The third edition presents an increased focus on occupation in all areas of documentation, and numerous references have been added throughout the text in an effort to present evidence-based information.

Two new chapters (Chapters 3 and 4) expand on information that was covered only briefly in previous editions. The contents of some chapters have been reorganized to make the material easier to understand, and the order of some chapters has been reorganized for a more logical presentation of the material. Several examples have been updated and added to reflect current practice in early intervention, mental health, seating and mobility, driver rehabilitation, work hardening, assistive technology, and community practice. There is also an increased focus of the impact of electronic documentation methods, with multiple examples provided.

Perhaps the most significant change in this edition is the introduction of a new format, called the COAST method (Chapter 6), for writing goals and objectives. This new format is intended to make goal writing less confusing and to improve the focus on occupation during the goal-writing process.

All worksheets presented in this manual will now be available on a Web site. This will give students the option of using either the perforated worksheets in the book or accessing them in an electronic version.

In addition to the changes listed above, this edition also comes with an Instructor's Manual that will be helpful to occupational therapy instructors teaching courses that involve documentation or fieldwork. The Instructor's Manual includes recommendations for use of the worksheets in the textbook, as well as suggestions for other assignments and quizzes. Grading rubrics are provided for evaluating student performance in writing functional problem statements, goals, intervention plans, and SOAP notes. The Instructor's Manual also includes access to videos that may be used for developing documentation skills. A case history and sample documentation accompany each video.

The Health Record

The health record, often called the *medical record*, is a compilation of data that includes the client's past and present health information. The purpose of the health record is to serve as the medical and legal document of a client's history, his or her current condition and status, the intervention provided, and the client's response to intervention (Hussey, Sabonis-Chafee, & O'Brien, 2007; Sames, 2009; Scott, 2006). Like many aspects of health care, the health record is continuously undergoing changes. Before moving on to the specific processes involved in documenting occupational therapy practice, it is important to understand the history of health records in general and the implications for occupational therapy documentation. This chapter will provide a brief history of health records in general, a history and overview of SOAP notes, and a discussion of the many audiences and functions of the health record.

HISTORY OF HEALTH RECORDS

The recording of patient information can be traced to the cave paintings and stone carvings of prehistoric times (Brodnik, 2007). As civilizations developed, people transitioned to the use of pen and paper for recording events. In the 1700s, ledgers were used to record information for various businesses in the United States including banks, stores, and eventually hospitals. Benjamin Franklin, secretary of one of the first incorporated hospitals in Pennsylvania in 1792, kept records of clients' names, addresses, disorders, and dates of admission and discharge. As medicine has advanced, so has the complexity and detail of the record. A profession, now called Health Information Management, was created to oversee the collection, classification, storage, retrieval, and dissemination of health records (American Health Information Management Association [AHIMA], 2009).

The use of computers to support health records management can be traced back to the late 1950s (Carter, 2008). Over the last few decades, the electronic health record (EHR) has gone from the exception to the rule. While the acceptance and use of EHRs has been slow and controversial, their use has the potential to streamline and improve the overall quality of client care, increase efficiency of health practitioners, and reduce health care costs (Baron, 2007; Ford, Menachemi, Peterson, & Huerta, 2009; Lohr, 2009). In 2004, President George W. Bush called for Universal EHR Adoption by 2014 (Ford et al., 2009; Scott, 2006). In 2009, President Barack Obama announced billions of dollars in financial support for health records technology to accelerate the use of EHRs nationwide (Lohr, 2009; O'Harrow, 2009).

HISTORY OF THE SOAP NOTE

EHRs allow members of a client's health care team to access information with a few simple clicks of the mouse. While many health care organizations have moved either fully or partially to EHRs, printed health records are

Gateley CA, Borcherding S. *Documentation Manual for Occupational Therapy: Writing SOAP Notes, 3rd Edition* (pp. 7-12)
© 2012 SLACK Incorporated

still in use in many settings. Printed health records can be source-oriented, integrated, or problem-oriented (Berger & Diamant, 2005). Source-oriented records are organized by discipline. Integrated records are organized in chronological order, with the most current information provided first. However, it is the problem-oriented medical record (POMR) that is the basis for the SOAP note format presented in this manual.

The POMR was introduced by Dr. Lawrence Weed in the 1960s to standardize physician and nursing documentation (Scott, 2006). Weed believed that the POMR format offered a more client-centered approach by focusing on the client's problems and the progress made toward solving those problems. As part of the more client-centered approach to documentation, Weed recommended that the progress note be organized into four sections including the client's own perception of the situation, which previously had been considered irrelevant. He used the acronym SOAP to define the four sections:

1. *"S" (Subjective)*: This section includes the client's report of his or her problems, limitations, and needs as well as the client's perception of treatment and progress. Typically, the subjective section of the progress note is brief. However, in an initial evaluation report, the "S" might be longer, since it will include the information obtained in the initial interview.

2. *"O" (Objective)*: This section contains the health professional's observation of the client's performance and the treatment provided. In an initial evaluation note, this section also includes all of the measurable, quantifiable, and observable data that were collected.

3. *"A" (Assessment)*: This section is the health professional's analysis and interpretation of the events reported in the subjective and objective sections. This section shows the practitioner's clinical reasoning. An initial evaluation contains the functional problem list and the client's rehabilitation potential. Subsequent progress notes will focus on one or more problems from that list as well as the progress made and rehabilitation potential.

4. *"P" (Plan)*: This section is the health professional's plan of what to do next, and it includes the anticipated frequency and duration of services. An initial evaluation includes a detailed intervention plan. Subsequent progress notes specify the planned focus for future sessions with the client.

For nearly 30 years, Weed's system was popular in hospitals and rehabilitation centers. Many facilities that still utilize printed health records have returned to a more source-oriented health record, containing sections for each discipline. Even so, the SOAP format of progress notes continues to be used worldwide by many occupational therapists, physical therapists, nurses, physicians, psychologists, and social workers (Gagan, 2009). It is viewed as a clear and concise way to document a client's health information.

It is important to remember that SOAP is just a format—an outline for organizing information. Any note can be written in this format, although some lend themselves to it better than others. An initial assessment can be quite lengthy when written in SOAP format because it will contain an occupational profile, prior level of functioning, a summary of functional problems, and the detailed intervention plan including long- and short-term goals. For this reason, many practice settings do not use the SOAP format for the initial evaluation report, but the facility may use the SOAP format for treatment and progress notes.

The SOAP format is an alternative to narrative notes, which tend to be disorganized and subjective. It forces the writer to look at all four aspects of the intervention session and to present the information in an orderly fashion. Practitioners who learn to use the SOAP format will be able to adapt their documentation skills to nearly any practice setting. A more detailed explanation of each section of the SOAP note is provided in Chapters 7 through 10.

Health Insurance Portability and Accountability Act

In 1996, Congress passed the Health Insurance Portability and Accountability Act (HIPAA) to ensure that employees could maintain health benefits when changing jobs (Scott, 2006). Another major provision of HIPAA was the establishment of federal standards for the security, use, and disclosure of a client's protected health information (PHI; U.S. Department of Health & Human Services, 2006). The HIPAA Privacy Rule, effective since 2003, prevents unauthorized disclosure of a client's PHI. Clients are also accorded several rights under HIPAA (Roach, Hoban, Broccolo, Roth, & Blanchard, 2006). These include the following:

✦ The right to view and obtain a copy of the health record.

✦ The right to request revision or omission of information in the health record that is incorrect.

✦ The right to know how health information is used and shared with others.

✦ The right to decide if PHI can be used for purposes of marketing and research.

✦ The right to authorize the release of health information to selected individuals.

✦ The right to file a complaint if it is believed that health information has been used in a way that violates the law.

HIPAA has several implications for occupational therapy practitioners. Health records should not be left open on a desk or up on a computer screen where they could be read by others, and client information should not be discussed in any area where it may be overheard by individuals not involved in the client's care (Sames, 2010). You should also have a clear understanding of the privacy safeguards that are in place at your place of employment and your role in ensuring compliance with HIPAA laws. For example, what procedure should you follow if a client asks for a copy of the health record? Is there a form that must be signed in order for you to discuss health information with a client's relative or friend? What should your response be if another client innocently asks, "What's wrong with that person over there?"

USERS AND USES OF THE HEALTH RECORD

The obvious purpose of the health record is to document a client's health information for future reference. It is important to consider the many potential audiences and functions of the health record whenever you make an entry into a client's record.

CLIENT CARE MANAGEMENT

The health record is one of the ways the treatment team communicates with each other about the day-to-day aspects of the client's care. Other occupational therapy practitioners and members of the interdisciplinary treatment team will read your notes in order to coordinate care. In your note, you share the results of your evaluation, report the client's progress toward established goals, and advise other members of the team of your plan for continuing care, all of which are important to the treatment team. Good documentation is particularly important in ensuring continuity of care in settings where a single client may encounter multiple occupational therapy practitioners during the rehabilitation process.

REIMBURSEMENT

The health record is the source for what services were provided, and thus, for what services may be billed. Third-party payers such as Medicare, Medicaid, and private insurance companies may review documentation, not only for frequency and duration, but also to determine if the services provided to the client are worth paying for. Documentation in the health record is the primary means of justifying reimbursement for intervention (Scott, 2006).

UTILIZATION REVIEW AND UTILIZATION MANAGEMENT

The health record may be used for purposes of determining whether services provided to a client are appropriate, medically necessary, and efficient according to the policies and procedures established by federal and state regulatory agencies. Freedman (2006) explained the distinction between *utilization review* and *utilization management*, two terms that are often used interchangeably but have different meanings. Utilization review is a review of the health record that occurs after services have been provided to a client. Utilization management involves the proactive processes that take place before and during a client's provision of health services. These processes may include discharge planning from an acute care hospital setting or precertification for an acute care or rehabilitation unit stay. The goals of both utilization review and utilization management are to ensure compliance of health care providers and organizations to regulatory standards and to use a client's funds for health care in the most cost-effective manner. In either situation, documentation of occupational therapy services may help determine whether a client's admission and continued treatment is necessary and appropriate.

THE LEGAL SYSTEM

The health record is a legal document that substantiates what occurred during a client's illness and treatment. Any entries made in the health record, whether in print or electronic format, become a part of that legal document and may be "subpoenaed and used as evidence in a variety of legal matters" (Erickson, McKnight, & Utzman, 2008, p. 22). If you as an occupational therapist have to appear in court to testify, you will be very glad that your documentation is clear, accurate, and thorough. Court cases often occur years after the event or intervention that is being contested. You may not even remember the event or the client. What you have written in the health record will provide you with the information you need in order to testify.

QUALITY IMPROVEMENT

Quality improvement (QI) is the continuous process of a health care entity's monitoring, assessing, and improving the quality of client services and outcomes (Scott, 2006.) Facilities may have a QI committee that is in charge of identifying and solving problems in client care. The health record is one of the primary sources of information used in the QI process. An example of a QI process is the review of occupational therapy documentation to determine whether practitioners were documenting a client's pain level according to hospital policy, followed by the implementation of measures to increase the compliance with the hospital policy.

ACCREDITATION

Health care settings that bill Medicare and/or Medicaid for services must be accredited by a state survey agency to ensure compliance with applicable laws and regulations (Centers for Medicare & Medicaid Services [CMS], 2009a). Some health care facilities voluntarily seek accreditation from private entities, such as the Joint Commission on Accreditation of Healthcare Organizations (JCAHO) and the Commission on Accreditation of Rehabilitation Facilities (CARF), in order to improve their professional reputation as a provider of quality health care (Clark & Bloom, 2006). JCAHO accredits hospitals, long-term care and assisted-living centers, and home health agencies. JCAHO's focus is on improving the processes and outcomes of client care. CARF accredits rehabilitation services on the basis of providing team-based client care that is individualized and responsive to client needs. In all cases, accreditation surveyors rely heavily on the review of client health records during the accreditation survey of a facility.

RESEARCH

The health record may also be used to provide data for research by a variety of individuals. Public health entities may use the health record to identify and document the incidence of certain medical conditions. Medical researchers may collect and analyze data from the health record to improve methods of disease and injury prevention (Engel, Henderson, Fergenbaum, & Colantonio, 2009). In recent years, there has been a move toward evidenced-based practice in occupational therapy (Crepeau et al., 2009a). Occupational therapy practitioners may use the health record to analyze client outcomes in order to determine the efficacy of specific therapeutic interventions.

EDUCATION

The health record may be used as a teaching tool. Students in various health care professions use the health record to gain information about a client's prior medical history and current clinical condition. An occupational therapy student may review the health record to learn about quality occupational therapy intervention or to gain a better understanding of the roles and interventions of other members of the client's health care team.

BUSINESS DEVELOPMENT

Management teams use the information contained in the health record to plan and market services provided by a facility. For example, are there enough referrals for outpatient occupational therapy driving evaluations to warrant the cost of purchasing expensive assessment equipment and providing specialized training for staff? Does the number of referrals for inpatient occupational therapy following total joint replacement signify the need for additional occupational therapy staffing on the orthopedic unit?

THE CLIENT

Another significant user of the health care record is the client. When you are documenting in the health record, always remember that the client owns the information and may choose to exercise his or her right to read what you have written. Walker, Ahern, Le, and Delbanco (2009) found that an increasing number of health care consumers expect full and timely access to their health records, particularly with the increased use of technology for documenting health care information.

A recent trend in the United States is the use of a Personal Health Record (PHR), which is an EHR maintained and controlled by the client rather than the provider (CMS, 2009d). While providers still maintain a health record on each client, the PHR allows the individual to keep health information in an organized fashion for personal reference and for ease of communication with health care providers. A client may choose to include information in his or her PHR about occupational therapy services you have provided.

ORGANIZATION OF THE HEALTH RECORD

The organization of paper health records will vary depending on the setting, but most health records have tabbed dividers clearly indicating the location of pertinent information. For example, an inpatient hospital setting may use the following dividers:

+ Admissions information
+ Insurance
+ Physician orders
+ History and physical
+ Physician progress notes
+ Nurse progress notes
+ Rehabilitation progress notes
+ Lab and radiology
+ Surgery and other procedures
+ Medications
+ Outside records
+ Discharge planning
+ Miscellaneous

A multidisciplinary outpatient clinic may have a different health record organization. For example:

+ Client information
+ Insurance
+ Physician orders
+ Physical therapy
+ Occupational therapy
+ Speech therapy
+ Outside records
+ Miscellaneous

Reimbursement, Legal, and Ethical Considerations

The previous chapter provided an overview of the various purposes and uses of the health record and the potential impacts on the documentation of occupational therapy practitioners. Some of those issues warrant further explanation and discussion. Since documentation is the primary means of justifying reimbursement for services (Scott, 2006), it is important for occupational therapy practitioners to understand various reimbursement systems and pertinent terminology. Practitioners must be aware of federal and state laws and regulations that impact reimbursement and documentation. It is also necessary to understand the impact of *Official Documents* of the American Occupational Therapy Association (AOTA) on documentation. In addition, it is important to consider the ethical implications that practitioners may encounter regarding the documentation of occupational therapy services. While reimbursement, legal, and ethical issues will vary considerably between practice settings, this chapter will provide a general foundation of information to guide documentation in occupational therapy practice.

SOURCES OF REIMBURSEMENT

Funding sources for reimbursement of occupational therapy services can be categorized as follows (Hussey et al., 2007):

+ Public sources funded through federal and state government, such as Medicare, Medicaid, schools, and early intervention programs
+ Private sources such as insurance companies, worker's compensation, and self-pay by the client
+ Service clubs, private foundations, and volunteer organizations

This section will focus on general documentation requirements related to reimbursement by public and private sources. You must keep in mind that funding sources are continuously revising regulations and guidelines and you must remain up to date on current documentation requirements. Your fieldwork supervisor or employer will be an important resource in helping you understand the documentation expectations related to reimbursement.

MEDICARE

Medicare is a federal insurance program managed by the CMS (U.S. Department of Health & Human Services, 2009). Medicare helps pay the health care costs of people over age 65 and individuals with long-term disabilities. Robinson (2007) explained that occupational therapy services covered under Medicare must be **medically necessary** and **skilled**. Medically necessary means that services are consistent with accepted standards of practice for the client's condition. Skilled means that the services provided require the decision making and highly complex competencies of an occupational therapist or occupational therapy assistant with a knowledge base of human functioning and occupational performance. Nonskilled services are those that are routine or maintenance types of therapy, both of which could be carried out by nonprofessional personnel or caregivers. In addition to being

Gateley CA, Borcherding S. *Documentation Manual for Occupational Therapy: Writing SOAP Notes, 3rd Edition* (pp. 13-22)
© 2012 SLACK Incorporated

medically necessary and skilled, services must be provided "within a reasonable frequency, intensity, and duration for the condition" and there must be "an expectation that the patient will improve in a reasonable amount of time" (Robinson, 2007, p. CE-6). Medicare benefits are divided into four types (CMS, 2009b; Robinson, 2007):

1. *Part A*: Covers inpatient hospitalization for acute care, rehabilitation, and psychiatric care; long-term care or critical access hospitals; and skilled nursing facilities (SNFs), home health care, and hospice.
2. *Part B*: Covers doctors' services and outpatient care (including occupational therapy); also covers services in SNFs once Part A benefits have been exhausted.
3. *Part C*: Also known as the Medicare Advantage Plan. Private insurance companies contract with Medicare to manage a beneficiary's Medicare benefits. Occupational therapists may have to communicate with plan providers for prior authorization of services or to ensure that they are a network provider for the beneficiary.
4. *Part D*: Medicare prescription drug coverage.

Medicare Part A

Reimbursement under Medicare Part A is based on a Prospective Payment System (PPS), meaning that payment rates are predetermined based on the client's initial diagnoses and presenting problems (CMS, 2009e; Robinson, 2007). The criteria and assessments used to determine payment rates vary depending on the setting. The length of time that Medicare Part A will pay for a client's health care also varies per setting. It is important for occupational therapy practitioners to have a general understanding of the reimbursement differences between settings because those differences impact the services you will be able to provide and bill for as well as the type of documentation that will be required. Listed next is a summary of reimbursement procedures for various settings covered by Medicare Part A.

Inpatient Hospitals

Medicare Part A benefits cover up to 90 days of inpatient hospitalization for each illness. Payment is based on diagnostic categories called diagnostic-related groups (DRGs), and a per diem rate is established for each case. That flat rate includes everything from room and board to medication to various services ordered by the physician, including occupational therapy (Robinson, 2007).

Inpatient Rehabilitation Facilities

Medicare Part A payments are based on case mix groups (CMGs). Clients are assigned to a CMG based on data reported on the Inpatient Rehabilitation Facility–Patient Assessment Instrument (IRF-PAI) which is filled at admission and discharge (CMS, 2010a). Included in the IRF-PAI is the Functional Independence Measure (FIM) instrument, which measures the client's level of independence in 18 functional activities (Robinson, 2007; Uniform Data System for Medical Rehabilitation [UDSMR], 2010). Occupational therapists play an important role in documenting a client's performance in activities of daily living (ADLs) and other functional activities, and this information is used to help determine the client's scores on the FIM instrument of the IRF-PAI.

Inpatient Psychiatric Facilities

Medicare Part A payments are based on a DRG that is determined by the client's diagnosed psychiatric condition and one or more of 17 co-morbidities (Robinson, 2007). Although there is no limit to psychiatric inpatient care received in general hospitals, Medicare currently limits payment for inpatient care in a specialty psychiatric hospital to 190 days in a lifetime (CMS, 2009c).

Skilled Nursing Facilities

Medicare Part A allows up to 100 days per illness, with beneficiary copayment required for days 21 through 100 (Robinson, 2007). SNFs use an assessment tool called the Minimum Data Set (MDS 2.0) to report data about the client's diagnosis, functional status, and time spent in therapy. Since payment is based partly on the amount of time spent in therapy, complete and accurate documentation by the occupational therapist is essential for appropriate reimbursement.

Home Health Care

Medicare Part A covers up to 100 home health visits per illness, and the plan of care must be recertified by a physician every 60 days (CMS, 2009b; Robinson, 2007). Payment rates are calculated using a tool called the Outcomes and Assessment Information Set (OASIS). Documentation from the occupational therapist may be used to help complete the OASIS.

Hospice

Medicare Part A covers services for individuals who have a terminal condition with a life expectancy of 6 months or less. Reimbursement is based on projected costs of care to be provided in the home and/or on an inpatient basis. Occupational therapy services under hospice are limited to "comfort, safety, quality of life issues, and caregiver education and training" (Robinson, 2007, p. CE-3).

Medicare Part B

Occupational therapy services are also covered under Medicare Part B benefits. Clients typically have a monthly premium for this supplemental medical coverage and a 20% copayment based on the Medicare-approved amount for the service (CMS, 2009b; Robinson, 2007). In addition, there is a "cap" on outpatient occupational therapy services, meaning that Medicare will not reimburse services beyond a set limit (CMS, 2009f).

MEDICAID

Medicaid is a health insurance program jointly funded by the federal government and each individual state (Social Security Administration, 2009). It covers individuals who have limited income and meet certain eligibility requirements. Medicaid is administered by each individual state. While all states must follow general federal guidelines, there is considerable variance between states in terms of which individuals are eligible for Medicaid and what services are covered. There may also be differences within a single state between services that are covered by Medicaid for adults versus children. Occupational therapists must become familiar with the Medicaid documentation and reimbursement guidelines for the state in which they are practicing.

SCHOOLS

Part B of the Individuals with Disabilities Education Act (IDEA) of 2004 requires schools to provide students with disabilities a free appropriate public education (FAPE) in the least restrictive environment (LRE). The law applies to students ages 3 through 21. Section 504 of the Rehabilitation Act of 1973 and Title II of the Americans with Disabilities Act of 1990 (ADA) prohibit schools from excluding a student with a disability from participating in educational activities. Occupational therapists may be asked to provide direct services to help a child meet his or her educational goals. They may also be asked to provide consultative services to help the school determine necessary modifications and accommodations. Schools use an Individualized Education Program (IEP) to document the student's educational needs, goals, and services (U.S. Department of Education, 2006). Documentation requirements vary from school to school, but the services provided must be relevant to the educational setting (Jackson, 2007).

EARLY INTERVENTION PROGRAMS

The Early Intervention Program for Infants and Toddlers with Disabilities (Part C of IDEA) is a federal grant program that assists states in operating a program of early intervention services for infants and toddlers ages birth through two years and their families. The program targets children who have a diagnosis associated with developmental delay and children who are deemed at risk for developmental delay. A major provision of Part C is that services are to be provided in a child's natural environment. These include the child's home and community settings that are typical for children without disabilities, such as preschools and day cares. Eligibility requirements vary between states based on each state's definition of "at risk" (Jackson, 2007; Stephens & Tauber, 2005). Each child served in an early intervention program will have an Individualized Family Service Plan (IFSP) that includes the "family's desired outcomes for the child and the services that will be provided to meet those outcomes" (Stephens & Tauber, 2005, p. 773). Occupational therapy is one of the many services that may be provided as part of the IFSP, and documentation requirements will vary among states.

PRIVATE INSURANCE

An individual may have private health insurance through his or her employer or through the employer of his or her spouse or parent. The cost of such plans is often subsidized by the employer. Some individuals purchase private health insurance because it is not available through an employer. There are many different private insurance plans with varying coverage, and there may be specific requirements that must be followed in order for the insurance company to pay for health care services. These requirements may include seeking health care from only particular providers considered "in network," getting "pre-authorization" or prior approval before seeing a health care provider, and limiting the number of visits per year to a particular type of provider (National Endowment for Financial Education, 2006). Many health care settings have individuals whose role is to deal with these insurance issues, but occupational therapists may have more direct involvement in the process in some settings. Documentation must meet the requirements of the individual practice setting, and there may be additional documentation required for a client's specific insurance plan.

WORKER'S COMPENSATION

Worker's compensation is a type of business insurance that covers the medical expenses and wages of employees who are injured on the job. Each state has different requirements for its worker's compensation program. Occupational therapy may be a service covered under the medical expenses of the program. When a client has worker's compensation as the funding source, therapeutic interventions and documentation should focus on improving the individual's capacity to return to work (King & Olson, 2009).

BILLING CODES

Occupational therapy practitioners will encounter multiple coding systems as part of their documentation and billing processes. These coding systems are intended to provide a standard language between health care providers and reimbursement sources for describing a client's diagnosis and the services provided (Graham et al., 2007). It should be noted that the coding systems described in this section are updated frequently, and practitioners must keep track of changes that may impact their documentation.

ICD-9 AND ICD-10 CODES

The World Health Organization (WHO) developed the *International Classification of Diseases* (ICD) as a coding system for signs, symptoms, injuries, diseases, and conditions. ICD-9 was published in 1977 and has been used in the United States for over 30 years to classify a client's diagnosis. WHO has since published the 10th revision of the coding system, ICD-10 (2009). The National Center for Health Statistics published a set of clinical modifiers (ICD-10-CM) to provide additional specificity to the coding system. At the time of this publication, health care entities are in the process of transitioning from the old classification system to the ICD-10-CM (Graham et al., 2007). The CMS set October 1, 2013 as the implementation deadline for the transition to ICD-10-CM code set (American Academy of Professional Coders, 2009). Listed below are just a few examples of ICD-10-CM codes that occupational therapy practitioners may encounter (WHO, 2009):

- ✦ F 20.0   Paranoid schizophrenia
- ✦ F 84.5   Asperger's syndrome
- ✦ G 35   Multiple sclerosis
- ✦ G 56.0   Carpal tunnel syndrome
- ✦ G 80.2   Spastic hemiplegic cerebral palsy
- ✦ S 72.0   Fracture of neck of femur (hip fracture)

CURRENT PROCEDURAL TERMINOLOGY CODES

Current Procedural Terminology (CPT) Codes are owned and copyrighted by the American Medical Association (AMA). The codes are a standardized listing of descriptive and identifying terms for reporting medical services and procedures. CMS adopted the use of CPT codes in 1983 as the mandatory system of coding services under Medicare Part B. Most managed care and private insurance companies now base their reimbursements on the CPT values established by CMS (Torrey, 2011). New CPT codes are published yearly. Some codes may be deleted and others added. It is the responsibility of each occupational therapy practitioner and employer to understand the current codes that may be assigned for services provided. Listed below are a few common codes that occupational therapy practitioners may use in the billing process (AMA, 2009). Please note that this list is not all-inclusive:

- ✦ 97003   Occupational therapy evaluation
- ✦ 97004   Occupational therapy re-evaluation

+ 97110   Therapeutic exercise
+ 97112   Neuromuscular re-education
+ 97530   Dynamic therapeutic activity
+ 97535   Self/care home management training
+ 97537   Community/work reintegration
+ 97542   Wheelchair management training
+ 97545   Work hardening/conditioning
+ 97760   Orthotic management/training
+ 97761   Prosthetic management/training

LEGAL, REGULATORY, AND ETHICAL GUIDELINES

Occupational therapy practitioners must be aware of legal, regulatory, and ethical standards that impact documentation. The AOTA publishes several *Official Documents* that guide occupational therapy practice and have direct implications on documentation. In addition, each state has a practice act that further regulates occupational therapy practice. This section will highlight the key points of several documents that impact the documentation of occupational therapy practitioners.

SCOPE OF PRACTICE

This document delineates the domain and process of occupational therapy practice and describes the educational and certification requirements for occupational therapy practitioners. Occupational therapy is defined as "the therapeutic use of everyday life activities (occupations) with individuals or groups for the purpose of participation in roles and situations in home, school, workplace, community, and other settings" (AOTA, 2010c). Documentation should demonstrate that the services provided to a client fall within the scope of practice for the occupational therapy profession. Furthermore, practitioners must abide by state laws for licensure, continuing education, and supervision. Such laws may impact the credentials included in a practitioner's signature on documentation and the type of documentation required to reflect that appropriate supervision has been provided during the delivery of services.

STANDARDS OF PRACTICE FOR OCCUPATIONAL THERAPY

This document defines the standards that must be met to practice as an occupational therapist or occupational therapy assistant (AOTA, 2010d). It outlines the education, examination, and licensure requirements for occupational therapy practitioners. The document goes on to clarify professional roles during the process of service delivery and states that documentation must meet the "time frames, formats, and standards established by practice settings, federal and state law, other regulatory and payer requirements, external accreditation programs, and AOTA documents" (AOTA, 2010d, p. 4).

GUIDELINES FOR SUPERVISION, ROLES, AND RESPONSIBILITIES DURING THE DELIVERY OF OCCUPATIONAL THERAPY SERVICES

This document outlines the roles, responsibilities, and supervision requirements of occupational therapists, occupational therapy assistants, and occupational therapy aides in the provision of occupational therapy services, including documentation practice (AOTA, 2009).

Occupational Therapists

Occupational therapists are considered autonomous practitioners, meaning they are independent with all aspects of service delivery, including documentation of the evaluation, intervention plan, intervention implementation, and outcomes. Occupational therapists initiate and direct the evaluation, interpret the data, develop and direct the intervention plan, modify or discontinue the intervention plan when appropriate, and interpret outcomes of a client's occupational performance. They collaborate with occupational therapy assistants by delegating selected assessments and interventions and exchanging information throughout the evaluation and intervention process. Documentation should reflect an occupational therapist's involvement throughout the delivery of occupational therapy services.

Occupational Therapy Assistants

Occupational therapy assistants must deliver services under the supervision of an occupational therapist. The amount of supervision that must be provided will vary depending on the state of practice and funding source. Occupational therapy assistants may contribute to the evaluation process by implementing assessments that have been delegated by the occupational therapist and providing verbal and written reports of the client's performance to the occupational therapist. They may collaborate with the occupational therapist during the development of the intervention plan. They are responsible for knowing the client's occupational therapy goals and targeted outcomes, and they provide written documentation and verbal report to the occupational therapist about the client's progress toward those goals and outcomes. Finally, occupational therapy assistants select, implement, and modify "therapeutic activities and interventions that are consistent with demonstrated competency levels, client goals, and the requirements of the practice setting" (AOTA, 2009, p. 801). Their accompanying documentation should reflect that all guidelines have been followed throughout the delivery of occupational therapy services.

Occupational Therapy Aides

Occupational therapy aides provide supportive nonskilled services specifically delegated by the occupational therapist or occupational therapy assistant. Ultimately, the occupational therapist is responsible for the use and actions of the aide, but aides may be supervised by the occupational therapy assistant. Aides may provide non–client-related tasks such as clerical, maintenance, and work area or equipment preparation. They may also perform routine client-related tasks under stable, predictable circumstances if they have previously demonstrated competence in the task. Occupational therapy practitioners must adhere to state and payer regulations when utilizing aides and documenting the services provided by an aide.

Occupational Therapy Students and Occupational Therapy Assistant Students

While not addressed in an *Official Document*, AOTA has issued clarification of the supervision requirements for students when occupational therapy services are billed under Medicare. The requirements vary by setting and are summarized below (AOTA, 2007d; Black & Eberhardt, 2005):
+ *Medicare Part A–Inpatient Hospitalization*: No specific CMS rules; state laws should be followed.
+ *Medicare Part A–SNF*: Services of an occupational therapy student and/or occupational therapy assistant student must be provided in line of sight of an occupational therapist.
+ *Medicare Part A–Hospice*: No specific CMS rules; state laws should be followed.
+ *Medicare Part A–Home Health*: The occupational therapist or occupational therapy assistant must be present in the home at the time that services are provided by a student.
+ *Medicare Part B–Outpatient/SNF*: No level of supervision is adequate for Medicare Part B reimbursement of student services. This means that if a student is present and in any way participating in the assessment and treatment of a client, the occupational therapist must be present at all times, direct the service, make all judgments, and be solely responsible for the service and documentation of services provided. The occupational therapist must not simultaneously be treating another client.

GUIDELINES FOR DOCUMENTATION OF OCCUPATIONAL THERAPY

This document articulates the purposes of documentation, explains different types of documentation, and lists the fundamental elements that should be present in all occupational therapy documentation. Documentation should occur any time occupational therapy services are provided to a client. The term *client* may be used to describe an individual, organization, or population as defined in the *Framework-II*. According to the *Guidelines for Documentation of Occupational Therapy*, "the purpose of documentation is to:
+ Articulate the rationale for provision of occupational therapy services and the relationship of this service to the client's outcomes
+ Reflect the occupational therapy practitioner's clinical reasoning and professional judgment
+ Communicate information about the client from the occupational therapy perspective
+ Create a chronological record of client status, occupational therapy services provided to the client, and client outcomes" (AOTA, 2008a, p. 684)

There are several different types of documentation that occur throughout the occupational therapy process of evaluation, intervention, and outcomes. They include the following:

+ Evaluation or screening report
+ Re-evaluation report
+ Intervention plan
+ Service contact report
+ Progress report
+ Transition plan
+ Discharge or discontinuation report (AOTA, 2008a)

The different types of documentation will be explained in more detail in Chapter 13. Regardless of the type of documentation, there are several essential elements that must be present in all documentation:

+ Client's full name and case number (if applicable)
+ Date and type of occupational therapy contact
+ Type of documentation; name of agency and department
+ Signature immediately after the documentation with practitioner's name and professional credentials
+ Countersignature of documentation by students and occupational therapy assistants in accordance with state and facility standards
+ Terminology and abbreviations acceptable to the setting
+ Correction of errors by drawing a single line through the error and initialing the correction
+ Adherence to professional standards of technology use for purposes of documentation
+ Compliance with legal and agency requirements for storage and disposal of records
+ Compliance with confidentiality standards (AOTA, 2008a)

OCCUPATIONAL THERAPY CODE OF ETHICS AND ETHICS STANDARDS

This document outlines the principles intended to promote and maintain high professional standards of conduct. It is intended to guide decision making when ethical issues arise. In simple terms, practitioners must always consider the implications of their decisions and actions on occupational therapy clients. The seven principles are summarized below:

1. *Principle 1—Beneficence*: Practitioners will demonstrate concern for the health and safety of their clients.
2. *Principle 2—Nonmaleficence*: Practitioners will not exploit or inflict harm on clients.
3. *Principle 3—Autonomy and Confidentiality*: Practitioners will collaborate with clients to determine goals, obtain informed consent for services, respect the client's right to refuse services, and protect all confidential information.
4. *Principle 4—Social Justice*: Practitioners will communicate the benefit of occupational therapy services and advocate to ensure that services are available in a fair and equitable manner to all potential recipients.
5. *Principle 5—Procedural Justice*: Practitioners will comply with laws and regulations that guide the profession.
6. *Principle 6—Veracity*: Practitioners will provide truthful, accurate information in all forms of communication and avoid communication that is false, fraudulent, or deceptive.
7. *Principle 7—Fidelity*: Practitioners will demonstrate respect, fairness, discretion, and integrity in all professional relationships and will act to ensure that breaches of the Code of Ethics are corrected and reported appropriately (AOTA, 2010a).

These ethical principles have many direct implications for documentation of occupational therapy services. An individualized evaluation and plan of care should be documented for each client, and the collaborative process between practitioner and client must be well documented. Documentation and accompanying billing must accurately reflect the services that were provided and must be in compliance with applicable laws, guidelines, and regulations. Documentation must include accurate credentials of the practitioner providing service and a description of appropriate levels of supervision during service delivery when applicable to comply with legal and facility guidelines. Documentation should not contain false information or fabricated data, and practitioners must keep documentation confidential at all times (AOTA, 2006b).

STATE PRACTICE ACTS

Each state regulates the practice of occupational therapy. State practice acts may address issues such as "scope of practice, supervision, continuing competence, unprofessional conduct, and licensure requirements" (Benemerito, 2000, p. 10). Each of these issues may have either direct or indirect implications on a practitioner's documentation, and it is the responsibility of each practitioner to know and abide by statutes that govern occupational therapy practice.

REIMBURSEMENT, LEGAL, AND ETHICAL ISSUES

When practitioners do not abide by all of the guidelines presented in this chapter that impact practice and documentation, they may encounter unfortunate reimbursement, legal, and ethical situations. In some cases, even those practitioners who consistently meet all guidelines still find themselves in unfortunate situations. Some of the common situations involving occupational therapy documentation will be discussed in this section.

REIMBURSEMENT DENIALS

Medicare and other reimbursement sources look at health care documentation with increasing scrutiny when determining whether billed services will be reimbursed. Appealing a reimbursement denial requires valuable time and resources. Denials can often be avoided by consistently providing thorough documentation that meets all necessary requirements. Brennan and Robinson (2006) summarized several "pitfalls" that may occur in the different types of occupational therapy documentation required by Medicare and most other payers, thus leading to potential reimbursement denials:

✦ Initial evaluations
  • Medical history is not sufficient to support the plan of care.
  • There is a lack of meaningful interpretation of objective data.
  • There is an insufficient description of the client's prior level of function to determine current functional loss.
✦ Plan of care and certification
  • The complexity of interventions described does not indicate that the skills of an occupational therapist or assistant are necessary.
  • The intervention plan is not modified when the client's progress is slower or faster than originally anticipated.
  • Anticipated date of goals and outcomes being met changes without justification.
  • Inadequate baseline function is provided to measure change and outcomes.
  • Client's score on a standardized test is used as an outcome measure rather than functional performance of an occupation.
✦ Treatment encounter note
  • Treatment minutes documented in the note are inconsistent with the billing codes submitted.
  • Frequency of treatment has changed from the initial plan of care but is not justified in the note.
  • Skilled treatment was changed between notes but not documented accordingly.
✦ Progress reports
  • Documentation lacks a description of specialized skills utilized that would indicate medical necessity.
  • Report does not adequately describe the client's current status in relation to functional goals.
  • Amount of therapy is excessive relative to the functional outcome.
  • Services provided are not consistent with the original plan of care and no explanation is given for the change.
  • Specific details are lacking about the activity and the body part(s) involved.
  • Not enough information is provided about the type of activity when billing for group therapy.

✦ Discharge summary
  • There is insufficient information about progress toward identified goals.
  • Client and caregiver education for functional carryover is not documented.
  • Documented interventions do not support medical necessity.
  • Skilled intervention and progress toward goals since the last progress note are not well explained.

BILLING FRAUD AND ABUSE

Scott (2006) defined fraud as "a false misrepresentation of a material fact, made with the intent to deceive" (p. 158). Billing practices that may constitute fraud include filing claims for services that were not rendered, billing with incorrect CPT codes to enhance reimbursement, and failing to document and bill accordingly when multiple clients were treated simultaneously. Erickson et al. (2008) distinguished abuse as unintentional billing errors resulting from poor awareness of proper procedures. Occupational therapy practitioners must be diligent in documenting and billing for their services appropriately to avoid claims of fraud and abuse.

MALPRACTICE AND OTHER LEGAL CLAIMS

Health care malpractice claims may result from professional negligence, breach of client-professional contractual promise, liability for defective equipment or products that cause injury, or intentional misconduct. From a legal perspective, the documentation that appears in a client's health record is often considered the best evidence of what transpired between the client and health care provider. It is essential that occupational therapy practitioners document client interactions accurately and completely. If an occupational therapy practitioner is found guilty of malpractice, he or she may face serious consequences, including monetary loss, loss of reputation, and state and/or federal punitive action including loss of license to practice (Scott, 2006).

ETHICAL DILEMMAS

Many occupational therapy practitioners will encounter ethical dilemmas involving their documentation at some point in their careers. For example, suppose it is time to provide a progress note to a client's insurance company to request authorization for additional outpatient visits. In your opinion, the client has made great progress and really does not need any additional services, but the client tells you that she hopes she can keep seeing you for a few more weeks so she can get even stronger. While you always have the client's best interests in mind, you should never falsify or withhold information about a client's performance in your documentation.

The issue of productivity expectations can also lead to ethical dilemmas. Productivity is measured by comparing the number of units or minutes billed to the number of hours worked (DiCarlo, 2008). Many settings have stringent productivity targets with the expectation that clients will be treated concurrently or in groups. While treating multiple clients simultaneously is not unethical, the services must be documented and billed appropriately. Occupational therapy practitioners may find themselves torn between meeting the productivity expectations of their employer and providing quality, individualized care to their clients. Slater (2006) reiterated that "occupational therapy practitioners have a legal and ethical responsibility to their clients, regardless of facility policies" (p. 17). She recommended that practitioners follow the *Guidelines to the Occupational Therapy Code of Ethics* (AOTA, 2006b) by first attempting to address potential ethical violations internally, and then consulting with appropriate regulatory agencies that have jurisdiction over occupational therapy practice.

General Guidelines for Documentation

The first three chapters of this book have detailed the importance of good documentation skills. The health record is a communication tool while the client is receiving services, but it is also the source for financial, legal, and clinical accountability. Occupational therapy documentation should always contain the following:

- ✦ What services were provided and when they were provided.
- ✦ What was said and what happened.
- ✦ How the client responded to the service provided.
- ✦ Why the skill of an occupational therapy practitioner was required rather than the services of an aide, a family member, or another professional.

Before you write anything in the record, make these assumptions:

- ✦ Someone else will have to read and understand what I write because I may be sick or out of town the next time this client needs to be treated.
- ✦ This entry I am about to make will be scrutinized by a third-party payer. If I were a Medicare reviewer, would I want to pay for the services I am about to record?
- ✦ My client will exercise his or her right to read this record.

As discussed in Chapter 3, it is critical to know your payment sources when documenting. Some payers are looking for different outcomes than others. With a Medicare client, you will discuss activities of daily living (ADLs) and write goals for self-care activities. With a workers' compensation case, you will write goals that are oriented to returning to work. In home health care, you may need to document that your client is unable to leave home to receive services or that education on safety issues was provided to the caregiver. With a child, you will need to focus on educationally relevant services identified in the Individualized Education Program (IEP).

It is essential to remember that your documentation is a reflection of your professional identity and abilities. It is also a reflection of your academic institution, your department, and occupational therapy as a profession. Unless they have witnessed you treating a client, your documentation may be the primary way that others form an impression about your skills and professionalism. This chapter will review general rules for documenting in the health record, guidelines for documenting special situations, considerations in electronic documentation, abbreviations and symbols for documentation, and common documentation errors.

GENERAL RULES FOR DOCUMENTING IN THE HEALTH RECORD

There are several rules that should always be followed when documenting in the health record (Borcherding & Morreale, 2007; Erickson et al., 2008; Sames, 2010; Scott, 2006):

- ✦ *Always use waterproof, nonerasable black ink*: This prevents smearing, erasing, or otherwise changing the health record.

Gateley CA, Borcherding S. *Documentation Manual for Occupational Therapy: Writing SOAP Notes, 3rd Edition* (pp. 23-36) © 2012 SLACK Incorporated

✦ *Correct errors*: Never use correction fluid or correction tape! It is considered an illegal alteration of the record. If you make an error in the health record, draw a single line through it, write your correction, and initial the change:

CG

Pt. able to dress lower body with ~~verbal cues~~ min Ⓐ using a reacher.

  • If you inadvertently write your note in the wrong client's chart, draw a single line through the entire entry and write "wrong chart" beside it with your signature.

  • If you need to add something after you have written and signed your note, write an addendum with the current date and time.

✦ *Be sure all required data is present*: The *Guidelines for Documentation in Occupational Therapy* (AOTA, 2008a) specify the content for each type of note you may be writing. This information will be covered in Chapter 13.

✦ *Be as concise as possible without leaving out pertinent data*: You will have limited time for documentation under today's productivity standards, and other busy professionals appreciate being able to read what you have written in the shortest time possible.

✦ *Sign and date every entry*: Some facilities and funding sources also require you to document the time of day or number of minutes that the client received services. The standard format is first name, middle initial, last name, and credentials. Notes by students must be co-signed by a supervising therapist, and in some settings, notes by occupational therapy assistants must be co-signed by the supervising occupational therapist.

✦ *Identify the client on every page of documentation*: In a written health record, every page must include the client's full name and other identifying information as required by the facility in indelible ink or in the form of a stamp.

✦ *Document in a timely manner*: It is best to document as soon after a session as possible. This allows for the best communication between team members. It also ensures that your recollection of events will be accurate.

  • If you encounter a situation in which you need to document a session that occurred on another date, you should document "Late entry for (date)" at the beginning of the note.

✦ *Use appropriate terminology for the recipient of services*: When referring to the persons who receive occupational therapy services, the terms *client, patient, consumer, resident, veteran, participant, individual, student, teacher, child, caregiver, employer,* or *family* may be used. Use the term that is considered most respectful for your practice setting.

✦ *Be prudent in using abbreviations*: Use only the abbreviations that are approved by your facility. This will be discussed in further detail later in this chapter.

✦ *Focus on the client's experience and leave yourself out*: Unless it is absolutely relevant, do not mention yourself in the note. It is not necessary to say, "Therapist provided caregiver with skilled instruction in assisting client with self-care." Simply say, "Caregiver received skilled instruction in assisting client with self-care." In the rare cases when it is necessary to mention yourself in the note, refer to yourself in the third person. Do not use "I" or "me." Instead use "the therapist," "the clinician," or "the OT." For example: "Client cursed and pushed therapist's hand away when physical assistance was provided for grooming task."

✦ *Always adhere to legal and ethical guidelines*: Be familiar with laws, regulatory guidelines, facility policies, and AOTA *Official Documents* that impact documentation.

✦ *Write legibly*: Others must be able to read and understand what you have written.

✦ *Always be accurate and objective*: Report what was actually observed and avoid judging or interpreting the observations other than in the assessment portion of your note.

✦ *In terms of fiscal and legal accountability, "If it's not documented, it didn't happen"*: No activity or contact is ever considered a service that has been provided until a clinical entry has been made in the health record.

✦ *Avoid spelling, grammar, and punctuation errors*: As previously stated, your documentation is a reflection of your skills and professionalism. Errors in documentation can also present safety concerns for your client if another professional misinterprets your documentation due to such errors.

✦ *Avoid "red-flag" words*: Words such as *continued* and *maintained* suggest that progress is not occurring and funding sources may not reimburse for those services.

DOCUMENTING SPECIAL SITUATIONS

Sames (2010) explained that any unusual situations should be documented. For example, suppose during your morning ADL session with a client that you observe pain and swelling of the lower leg (symptoms of a blood clot) or a decrease in cognition from previous sessions. Those symptoms should be documented in the health record. It is also important to communicate any status change to the client's nurse and/or physician and to document that you have passed the information on to the appropriate person.

Another special situation that should be documented is a client's lack of compliance with medical and therapy recommendations. For example, if a client is not following safety recommendations, such as hip precautions or the use of an assistive device for ambulation during ADLs, it is important to document these observations along with any reasons that the client may provide for choosing not to follow the recommendations. It is, however, necessary to distinguish between voluntary lack of compliance and cognitive deficits that limit the client's ability to remember to comply with recommendations.

Any scheduled or attempted visits that are missed should be documented with an explanation for the missed visit and any other pertinent information regarding follow-up:

✦ *Client cancelled scheduled outpatient visit due to inclement weather. Confirmed next appointment on 12-1-2011.*

✦ *Attempted twice this date to see pt. for initial OT eval. Pt. off unit to diagnostic testing (TEE) in am, then on bed rest this pm following sedation from test. Will reattempt tomorrow.*

✦ *Resident declined participation in therapeutic exercise this am, citing fatigue. Rescheduled for this pm.*

✦ *Child missed two scheduled OT sessions on 11/1 & 11/3 due to being absent from school 11/1 – 11/4/2011 with illness. Will resume 30 minute sessions 2X/wk next week.*

✦ *Attempted scheduled home visit for early intervention. Child and family not home at scheduled time/date. Attempted twice to contact by phone, no answer, left message on voicemail. Notified service coordinator of situation.*

Another special situation that requires documentation is an incident report. An incident report should be completed for events such as client falls, skin tears, inadvertent removal of IV or catheter, and other unplanned events that led to injury or had the potential to lead to the injury of a client, visitor, or staff person. Scott (2006) reiterated that the incident report should **not** be contained in the health record, as it contains administrative information about follow-up of the incident. The health record should contain only the objective clinical information related to the event. For example, *"Client experienced ½-inch skin tear to dorsal aspect of (L) hand when reaching into kitchen cabinet during cooking activity. Pressure and gauze bandage applied; nursing notified. Client stated, 'I'm fine' and continued with cooking activity."* Health care settings have special forms and procedures for documenting incident reports, and such reports serve the following purposes:

✦ Ensuring that optimal care was provided to the injured party.

✦ Protecting the staff member and facility from unwarranted liability exposure.

✦ Identifying the need for further staff training to prevent similar incidents.

An incident involving injury to you will require additional documentation because it is considered a workers' compensation issue. Examples include injuring your back while transferring a client, slipping on a wet floor in a client's room, or being struck or bitten by a client. When any event occurs that would require an incident report, it is essential that you notify your supervisor immediately so that appropriate responses can be carried out and documented.

PEOPLE-FIRST LANGUAGE

Snow (2009) suggests that professionals should make an intentional effort always to refer to the individual first rather than the diagnosis. For example, rather than "the Down baby," we should say "the infant with Down syndrome." Rather than "the stroke patient," we should say "the patient who had a stroke."

This concept of people-first language fits well within our profession. One of the guiding principles for the occupational therapy profession is client-centered practice (Crepeau et al., 2009a). One way to demonstrate client-centered practice is by using people-first language not just in our verbal interactions, but also in our documentation. We should write our notes in terms of what the client needs rather than stating that the client **is** a particular assist level. Our clients are much more than their assist levels.

Please say: *"Veteran needs max assist…"* or *"Veteran requires max assist…"*
Rather than *"Veteran is max assist…"*

Considerations in Electronic Documentation

While electronic health records (EHRs) provide many advantages in terms of efficiency, connectivity, and legibility, they also present unique concerns, particularly in regard to confidentiality. The HIPAA Security Rule established federal standards for the security of EHRs. All employees who have access to EHRs must take precautions to prevent unauthorized access, alteration, or disclosure of a client's health information (Roach et al., 2006; Scott, 2006). Occupational therapy practitioners who have access to EHRs will generally have a username and/or password to access client records and to sign documentation that has been entered about occupational therapy services. The following precautions should be taken to adhere to the HIPAA Security Rule:

✦ Do not share your username or password with anyone.

✦ Logout when you are leaving an electronic workstation.

✦ Do not access any EHRs that you do not have a direct need to see. This includes your own EHR or those of family, friends, etc. Access to unauthorized EHRs can be traced back to your username and may be grounds for disciplinary action, termination of employment, and legal action.

✦ Be aware of your surroundings and make sure that unauthorized individuals cannot read the screen. Electronic workstations are often located in high traffic areas such as nurses' stations, patient rooms, hallways, therapy gyms, and shared offices.

✦ Be familiar and compliant with your employer's EHR safeguards, including the transmission of personal health information (PHI) via facsimile or electronic mail.

While EHRs increase legibility of documentation, they do not eliminate the potential for errors. Many programs have a spell check feature to reduce spelling errors, but such programs may not catch typographical errors such as the reversal of letters resulting in a different, correctly spelled word. Occupational therapy practitioners should carefully review what they have entered into an EHR prior to providing an electronic signature.

Avoiding Common Documentation Errors

As previously stated, your documentation is a reflection of you and the profession of occupational therapy. Mistakes in spelling, grammar, and punctuation may give others a negative impression of your knowledge, skills, and professionalism. Such errors can also lead to serious consequences for you or your client. This section will review several rules to help you avoid common documentation errors (Borcherding & Morreale, 2007; Villemaire & Villemaire, 2001):

✦ Use quotation marks when documenting the exact words that a client or another person said.
  • Incorrect: *Client stated I can't feel my right arm.*
  • Correct: *Client stated, "I can't feel my right arm."*

✦ Do not use quotation marks when paraphrasing what a client or another person said.
  • Incorrect: *Client reports she "can't feel her right arm."*
  • Correct: *Client reports she cannot feel her right arm.*

✦ Be consistent in use of verb tense.
  • Incorrect: *Client demonstrated upper body dressing with min Ⓐ. Client threads Ⓡ UE into sleeve first. Client transfers to toilet with SBA. Client completed grooming tasks independently.*
  • Correct: *Client demonstrated upper body dressing with min Ⓐ. Client threaded Ⓡ UE into sleeve first. Client transferred to toilet with SBA. Client completed grooming tasks independently.*

✦ Indicate plurals by adding an "s" to the end of a word **without** an apostrophe.
  • Incorrect: *The client's participated in a group discussion about time management and ADL's. The OT's then provided additional suggestion's.*
  • Correct: *The clients participated in a group discussion about time management and ADLs. The OTs then provided additional suggestions.*

✦ Indicate possession of a **single** person or object by using an apostrophe **before** the "s."
  - Incorrect: *The clients' spouse was present during the session.*
  - Correct: *The client's spouse was present during the session.*
✦ Indicate possession of **more than one** person or object by using and apostrophe **after** the "s."
  - Incorrect: *The three clients group discussion focused on coping skills.*
  - Correct: *The three clients' group discussion focused on coping skills.*
✦ Use a singular pronoun to refer to one person.
  - Incorrect: *The client has difficulty putting on their shirt.*
  - Correct: *The client has difficulty putting on his shirt.*
✦ Use a plural pronoun to refer to more than one person.
  - Incorrect: *They blame themself for the situation.*
  - Correct: *They blame themselves for the situation.*
✦ Follow the general rules for capitalization (Table 4-1).
✦ Know the appropriate spelling of commonly misspelled words (Table 4-2).

Table 4-1

General Rules for Capitalization

CAPITALIZE	DO NOT CAPITALIZE
Proper names in medical terminology ◆ e.g., Asperger's syndrome	Common nouns in medical terminology ◆ e.g., virus, appendectomy, scapula
Trade names of products and medications ◆ e.g., Jobst stocking, Ibuprofen	Generic drugs and products ◆ e.g., compression glove, pain reliever
Specific Organizations ◆ e.g., Joint Commission on the Accreditation of Healthcare Organizations (JCAHO)	Generic organizations ◆ e.g., accrediting agency
Academic degrees and professional designations after the person's name ◆ e.g., Crystal Gateley, MA, OTR/L	General degrees or generic professional designations ◆ e.g., an associate's degree, an occupational therapist
Exact test titles ◆ e.g., Peabody Developmental Motor Scales	Generic test ◆ e.g., sensory test, cognitive test
Specific department proper names ◆ e.g., Midwest Hospital Occupational Therapy Department	Generic department names ◆ e.g., an occupational therapy department, the rehab department
Official titles as part of a name ◆ e.g., Dr. McCormack, Father O'Malley	Generic or descriptive titles ◆ e.g., the doctor, the clergyman

Information compiled from Borcherding, S., & Morreale, M. (2007). *The OTA's guide to writing SOAP notes.* Thorofare, NJ: SLACK Incorporated.; Villemaire, D., & Villemaire, L. (2001). *Grammar and writing skills for the health professional.* Albany, NY: Delmar.

Table 4-2

Commonly Misspelled Words

Words That Sound Alike	"I" Before "E", Except After "C" Words	Miscellaneous Words
• accept (*She wouldn't accept it.*) • except (*all except that one*) • affect (*He had a flat affect. That didn't affect his participation.*) • effect (*That has no effect on me.*) • aid (*verb—to help; noun—a helping device, such as a "visual aid"*) • aide (*person, such as the OT aide*) • brake (*Lock the wheelchair brake.*) • break (*Take a break. He will break his arm.*) • gait (*ambulation*) • gate (*an entrance*) • lay (*Lay it on the desk.*) • lie (*He wants to lie on the bed.*) • loose (*not tight*) • lose (*I want to lose weight.*) • peace (*I want some peace and quiet.*) • piece (*piece of the puzzle*) • principal (*the school principal*) • principle (*principles of NDT*) • stationary (*not moving*) • stationery (*writing paper*) • than (*I have more than you.*) • then (*Then he went to bed.*) • their (*It was their house.*) • there (*Put it there.*) • they're (*they are*) • wait (*Wait here.*) • weight (*Her weight has declined.*) • you're (*you are*) • your (*It's your turn.*)	• achieve (after "ch" is still "ie") • believe • brief • hygiene • receive • relieve • retrieve	• activity • Alzheimer's • asymmetry • catheterization • clavicle • current • deferred • definitely • developmentally • dining • doctor • doff • doffed • doffing • dominant • don • donned • equilibrium • exercise • immobilize • independent • input • interest • judgment • paraffin • perform • putty • remember • rotator cuff • schizophrenia • stabilization • symmetry • technique • tolerate • transferring • writing

Information compiled from Borcherding, S., & Morreale, M. (2007). *The OTA's guide to writing SOAP notes.* Thorofare, NJ: SLACK Incorporated.; Merriam-Webster. (2003). *Merriam-Webster's collegiate dictionary* (11th ed.). Springfield, MA: Author..

ABBREVIATIONS AND SYMBOLS

Using abbreviations and symbols when documenting in the client's health record saves valuable time, but these should be used with discretion (Scott, 2006). Remember that your notes may be read by someone who knows little about occupational therapy, and that individual may determine whether to pay for your services or not. You should be sure that the individual will be able to understand the information you are trying to convey. Health care settings typically have a list of approved abbreviations. You should be familiar with that list and use only abbreviations that are approved for your setting. Do not make up abbreviations. Many people commonly use acronyms or shorthand when chatting online or texting, but those abbreviations are not appropriate for the health record. Also remember that while it is **permissible** to use abbreviations, it is not **required**. You may write out any word instead of shortening it. In this manual, you will find that some notes use more abbreviations and symbols than others. Table 4-3 lists commonly used abbreviations.

The Joint Commission on the Accreditation of Health Care Organizations (JCAHO), which accredits many hospitals and other health care facilities, does not maintain a list of acceptable abbreviations and symbols for use in documentation. JCAHO has published an *Official "Do Not Use" List of Abbreviations* (JCAHO, 2009). The list contains abbreviations and symbols prohibited on all orders and handwritten, pre-printed, and electronic forms regarding medications and can be found at www.jointcommission.org. A few examples of prohibited abbreviations are Q.D. (every day) and Q.O.D. (every other day) because they can be mistaken for each other. While occupational therapy practitioners would rarely have involvement with documentation regarding medications, some facilities prohibit the use of the abbreviations and symbols on the *Do Not Use List* by any health care provider in any type of documentation. You must be familiar with the list of acceptable and prohibited abbreviations and symbols for your facility.

Table 4-3

Abbreviations and Symbols

ABBREVIATIONS FOR DIAGNOSES, PROCEDURES, AND BODY PARTS

AAA	abdominal aortic aneurysm	A/P	anterior/posterior	CAT	computerized axial tomography
Ⓐ	assistance	ARF	acute renal failure	cath.	catheter; catheterization
A&Ox4	alert and oriented to person, place, time, situation	ASCVD	atherosclerotic cardiovascular disease	CBC	complete blood count
$\bar{a}$	before	ASHD	arterial sclerotic heart disease	c-diff	*C. difficile* (bacteria)
abd	abduction			CF	cystic fibrosis
ABG	arterial blood gas	ASIS	anterior superior iliac spine	chemo	chemotherapy
add	adduction			CHF	congestive heart failure
ADD	attention deficit disorder	Ⓑ	bilateral	CHI	closed head injury
ADHD	attention deficit hyperactivity disorder	BE	below elbow	CMC	carpometacarpal
		Bi-PAP	bi-level positive airway pressure	CNS	central nervous system
AE	above elbow	BK	below knee	C/O	complains of
AIDS	acquired immunodeficiency syndrome	BKA	below knee amputation	CO$_2$	carbon dioxide
		BM	bowel movement	COPD	chronic obstructive pulmonary disease
AK	above knee	BP	blood pressure	CP	cerebral palsy
AKA	above knee amputation	BRP	bathroom privileges	CPAP	continuous positive airway pressure
ALS	amyotrophic lateral sclerosis	$\bar{c}$	with		
		CA	cancer; carcinoma	CPM	continuous passive motion (machine)
AMA	against medical advice	CABG	coronary artery bypass graft		
ant.	anterior			CPR	cardiopulmonary resuscitation
appt.	appointment	CAD	coronary artery disease		

(continued)

Table 4-3 (continued)

Abbreviations and Symbols

ABBREVIATIONS FOR DIAGNOSES, PROCEDURES, AND BODY PARTS

CRF	chronic renal failure	HIV	human immunodeficiency virus	OA	osteoarthritis
CSF	cerebrospinal fluid	HOH	hard of hearing	ORIF	open reduction internal fixation
CT	computed tomography	H&P	history and physical	$\bar{p}$	after
CTR	carpal tunnel release	HR	heart rate	PCA	patient controlled analgesia
CVA	cerebrovascular accident	HTN	hypertension		
CXR	chest x-ray	Hx	history	PCA	personal care attendant
DDD	degenerative disk disease	I&D	incision and drainage	PDD	pervasive developmental disorder
DIP	distal interphalangeal joint	IM	intramuscular	PEG	percutaneous endoscopic gastrostomy
		I&O	intake and output		
DJD	degenerative joint disease	IV	intravenous	peri.	perineal
DM	diabetes mellitus	Ⓛ	left	PET	positron emission tomography
DNR	do not resuscitate	LLQ	left lower quadrant		
DOB	date of birth	LMN	lower motor neuron	PIP	proximal interphalangeal joint
DTR	deep tendon reflex	LOC	loss of consciousness		
DVT	deep vein thrombosis	LP	lumbar puncture	PMH	previous medical history
Dx	diagnosis	LUQ	left upper quadrant	PNS	peripheral nervous system
ECG	electrocardiogram	MCP	metacarpalphalangeal		
ECHO	echocardiogram	MD	muscular dystrophy; medical doctor	PO	by mouth; orally
EEG	electroencephalogram			postop	postoperatively
EKG	electrocardiogram	meds.	medications	preop	preoperatively
EMG	electromyogram	mets.	metastases	PSIS	posterior superior iliac spine
ENT	ear, nose, throat	MI	myocardial infarction		
EOM	extraocular movement	MP	metacarpophalangeal joint	PVD	peripheral vascular disease
ESRD	end stage renal disease	MRA	magnetic resonance angiogram	Ⓡ	right
EtOH	ethanol (alcohol use/abuse)			RA	rheumatoid arthritis
		MRI	magnetic resonance imaging	RBC	red blood cell count
FBS	fasting blood sugar			RLQ	right lower quadrant
FTT	failure to thrive	MRSA	Methicillin-resistant *Staphylococcus aureus* (bacteria)	R/O	rule out
F/U	follow-up			RSD	reflex sympathetic dystrophy
Fx	fracture	MS	multiple sclerosis		
GB	gall bladder	MVA	motor vehicle accident	RTC	return to clinic
GERD	gastroesophageal reflux disease	NC	nasal cannula	RTO	return to office
		NG	nasogastric (tube)	RUQ	right upper quadrant
GI	gastrointestinal	NKA	no known allergies	Rx	prescription
GSW	gunshot wound	NKDA	no known drug allergies	$\bar{s}$	without
H/A	headache	NOS	not otherwise specified	SCI	spinal cord injury
HEENT	head, eyes, ears, nose, throat	NPO	nothing by mouth	SDH	subdural hematoma
		N/V	nausea and vomiting	SLE	systemic lupus erythematosus
		O_2	oxygen	SOB	shortness of breath

(continued)

Table 4-3 (continued)

Abbreviations and Symbols

ABBREVIATIONS FOR DIAGNOSES, PROCEDURES, AND BODY PARTS

S/P	status post	THR	total hip replacement	URI	upper respiratory infection
S/S	signs and symptoms	TIA	transient ischemic attack		
Sx	symptoms	TKA	total knee arthroplasty	US	ultrasound
Sz	seizure	TKR	total knee replacement	UTI	urinary tract infection
TB	tuberculosis	tPA	tissue plasminogen activator	VRE	Vancomycin-resistant *enterococci* (bacteria)
TBI	traumatic brain injury				
TEDS	thromboembolic disease stockings	TPN	total parenteral nutrition	WBC	white blood cell count
		Tx	treatment	Wt	weight
TEE	transesophageal echo-cardiogram	UA	urinalysis	y.o.	year old
		UMN	upper motor neuron	yr.	year
THA	total hip arthroplasty				

ABBREVIATIONS FOR FREQUENCY AND TIME

ad lib	as desired	PTA	prior to admission	1x/wk	once a week
AM	morning	qd	every day	2x/wk	twice a week
ASAP	as soon as possible	qid	four times a day	3x/wk	three times a week
bid	twice a day	qod	every other day	1x/mo	once a month
noc	night or bedtime	STAT	immediately	2x/mo	twice a month
PM	afternoon	tid	three times a day	3x/mo	three times a month
prn	as needed				

ABBREVIATIONS FOR LOCATION AND SETTINGS

CCU	coronary (cardiac) care unit	LTC	long-term care	PICU	pediatric intensive care unit
		MICU	medical intensive care unit		
ECF	extended care facility			RCF	residential care facility
ED	emergency department	NICU	neonatal intensive care unit	SICU	surgical intensive care unit
ER	emergency room				
HH	home health	OP	outpatient	SNF	skilled nursing facility
ICU	intensive care unit	OR	operating room	SNU	skilled nursing unit
IP	inpatient	PACU	post-anesthesia care unit		

ABBREVIATIONS FOR LEVELS OF ASSISTANCE

Ⓘ	independent	Min Ⓐ	minimal assistance	Ⓓ	dependent assistance
Mod Ⓘ	modified independent	Mod Ⓐ	moderate assistance	x1	assistance of 1 person
SBA	stand by assistance	Max Ⓐ	maximal assistance	x2	assistance of 2 people
CGA	contact guard assistance				

MISCELLANEOUS COMMON THERAPY ABBREVIATIONS

AAROM	active assistive range of motion	amb.	ambulation; ambulated	BADLs	basic activities of daily living
		AROM	active range of motion		
ADLs	activities of daily living	ATNR	asymmetrical tonic neck reflex	CHT	certified hand therapist
AFO	ankle foot orthosis				

(continued)

Table 4-3 (continued)

Abbreviations and Symbols

MISCELLANEOUS COMMON THERAPY ABBREVIATIONS

COTA	certified occupational therapy assistant	KAFO	knee ankle foot orthosis	Pt.	patient
COTA/L	certified occupational therapy assistant/ licensed	LE	lower extremity	PTA	physical therapist assistant
		LOS	length of stay	PWB	partial weightbearing
		MMT	manual muscle testing	rehab	rehabilitation
CST	craniosacral therapist	N	normal (muscle grade)	SI	sensory integration
D/C	discontinue; discharge	NDT	neurodevelopmental treatment	SLP	speech language pathologist
DME	durable medical equipment	NMES	neuromuscular electrical stimulation	SOAP	subjective, objective, assessment, plan
ELOS	estimated length of stay	NWB	non-weightbearing	SOC	start of care
EOB	edge of bed	OOB	out of bed	STG	short-term goal
e-stim	electrical stimulation	OT	occupational therapist; occupational therapy	STM	short-term memory
eval.	evaluation			STNR	symmetrical tonic neck reflex
ext.	extension	OTR	occupational therapist, registered		
F	fair (muscle grade)			TDWB	touch down weightbearing
FIM	Functional Independence Measure	OTR/L	occupational therapist, registered/licensed		
flex.	flexion	OTS	occupational therapy student	TENS	transcutaneous electrical nerve stimulation
ft.	foot; feet				
FWB	full weightbearing	P	poor (muscle grade)	TTWB	toe touch weightbearing
G	good (muscle grade)	PAM	physical agent modality	UE	upper extremity
HEP	home exercise program	PLOF	prior level of function	WBAT	weightbearing as tolerated
HOB	head of bed	PNF	proprioceptive neuromuscular facilitation		
HOH	hand over hand			w/c	wheelchair
IADLs	instrumental activities of daily living	POC	plan of care	WFL	within functional limits
		PT	physical therapist; physical therapy	WNL	within normal limits
IEP	Individualized Education Program				

MISCELLANEOUS SYMBOLS

♀	female	'	feet	~	approximately
♂	male	°	degree	%	percent
↓	decrease	+	plus, positive	&	and
↑	increase	–	minus, negative	@	at
c̄	with	#	number (#1); pounds	↔	to and from
s̄	without	/	per	→	to; progressing toward
ā	before	<	less than	1°	primary
p̄	after	>	greater than	2°	secondary; due to
"	inches	=	equals		

Information compiled from Borcherding, S., & Morreale, M. (2007). *The OTA's guide to writing SOAP notes*. Thorofare, NJ: SLACK Incorporated.; Chabner, D. (2004). *Medical language instant translator* (2nd ed.). St. Louis, MO: Elsevier.; Myers, T. (Ed.). (2009). *Mosby's dictionary of medicine, nursing & health professions*. St. Louis, MO: Mosby/Elsevier.; Sames, K. (2010). *Documenting occupational therapy practice* (2nd ed.). Upper Saddle River, NJ: Pearson.; Scott, R. (2006). *Legal aspects of documenting patient care for rehabilitation professionals*. Sudbury, MA: Jones and Bartlett Publishers.

WORKSHEET 4-1

Avoiding Common Documentation Errors

Identify and correct the errors in the following statements.

1. Pt. stated my head really hurts this morning.

2. Resident reported "her right hand is working better today."

3. Student used right hand to cut with scissors. Student then switches to left hand for coloring tasks. Student did not demonstrate consistent hand preference.

4. The client's expressed excitement about the upcoming visit to the mall.

5. An occupational therapy referral was recieved from the childs' teacher.

6. The child was unable to button their coat.

7. The resident's were all in the dinning room weighting for there meal.

8. Client demonstrated appropriate social interaction by responding your welcome to another group member.

9. Pt. required moderate assistance to use dominate right hand in hygeine tasks.

10. Client does not demonstrate awareness of the affect of his mood on other member's of the group.

11. Pt. expressed intrest in getting dressed. Pt required verbal cues when doning pullover shirt to utilize adaptive teckniques due to right rotary cup injury.

Worksheet 4-1 (continued)
Avoiding Common Documentation Errors

Identify and correct the errors in the following statements.

12. The ot noticed assymetry in the childs sitting posture. Parents reports that the client is unable to sit independantly.

13. The OTR preformed a Cognitive Test on the client.

14. The Doctor called to check on the Patients status.

15. Client demonstrated poor judgement by attempting to stand up without their walker.

16. Pt. had right arm imobilized due to a clavical fracture.

17. Client required several breif rest brakes during ADL's.

18. The clinic employs three otr's and two ota's.

19. The students principle stated Jimmy is disruptive at school.

20. A child at this age should be able to dress themselves.

21. The childrens' mother has difficulty keeping all they're appointment's.

22. Client needed a visual aide to help them learn how to preform self-catherization.

Worksheet 4-2

Using Abbreviations

Translate each sentence written with abbreviations into full English phrases or sentences.

1. Client c/o pain in Ⓡ MCP joint p̄ ~15 min PROM.

2. Pt. A&OX4.

3. Client transferred w/c → mat c̄ sliding board & max Ⓐ X 2.

4. 1° dx Ⓛ BKA, 2° dx COPD, CHF, DM, & PVD.

5. Pt. is s/p Ⓡ THR. Orders received for OT 2x/day for ADLs & IADLs, TTWB Ⓡ LE.

Shorten these sentences using only the standard abbreviations in this chapter.

6. Client has thirty degrees of passive range of motion in the left distal interphalangeal joint, which is within functional limits.

7. Client is able to put on her socks with standby assistance, but requires moderate assistance with putting on and taking off left shoe.

8. The client requires contact guard assistance for balance during her morning dressing, which she performs while sitting on the edge of her bed.

WORKSHEET 4-2 (CONTINUED)
Using Abbreviations

Shorten these notes using only the standard abbreviations in this chapter.

9. The patient participated in a bedside evaluation of activities of daily living. She was able to perform bed mobility with moderate assistance, but she needed maximum assistance to put on her adult undergarment. She was able to go from a supine position to a sitting position with minimum assistance and from a sitting position to a standing position with moderate assistance.

10. The resident came to the occupational therapy clinic via wheelchair escort. The resident was observed to lean toward his left. The resident needed verbal cues and minimum assistance in positioning his body in the wheelchair to maintain midline orientation and symmetrical posture. The resident transferred from his wheelchair to the toilet with moderate assistance of one person to help him keep his balance using a standing pivot transfer. He needed verbal cues and visual feedback from a mirror to maintain upright posture.

11. The veteran participated in an evaluation in his room to determine relevant client factors. The veteran's short-term memory was three out of three for immediate recall, one out of three after 1 minute, and zero out of three with verbal cues after 5 minutes. The left upper extremity shoulder flexion was a grade of 4, shoulder extension was a grade of 4, elbow flexion was a grade of 4, elbow extension was a grade of 4, wrist flexion was a grade of 4 minus, wrist extension was a grade of 4 minus, and grip strength was 8 pounds. The left upper extremity light touch was intact. The right upper extremity muscle grades and sensation were within functional limits.

Writing Functional Problem Statements

As a part of the initial assessment, the occupational therapist develops a "problem list" identifying the major areas of occupation that have been impacted by the client's condition. The contributing factors that affect the client's occupational performance are also identified. Priorities are then set with the client and caregivers so that the problems that are most important to them will be addressed. Some clients may need clarification of occupational therapy's role in order to identify problem areas that fall within the scope of occupational therapy practice. Educating the client about the purpose and potential benefits of occupational therapy is an important part of establishing a therapeutic relationship (Price, 2009). Clients that take an active role in goal setting often have improved functional outcomes and report greater satisfaction with the rehabilitation process (Tripicchio, Bykerk, Wegner, & Wegner, 2009).

There are two parts to a functional problem statement: the area of occupation that is a concern, and the contributing factors that are interfering with the client's engagement in that area of occupation. Let's take a closer look at information that was presented in Chapter 1 about occupational therapy's domain.

AREAS OF OCCUPATION

Occupational therapy practitioners provide interventions for people who have problems engaging in an area of occupation. This is important to note because this is what we will document. The focus on ability to engage in occupation is what distinguishes the occupational therapy profession from other health care disciplines. The *Occupational Therapy Practice Framework: Domain & Process, 2nd Edition* (AOTA, 2008b) categorizes the areas of occupation (Table 5-1) that may be addressed by occupational therapy practitioners.

It is essential to remember that the entities and agencies that provide reimbursement for occupational therapy services have differing priorities. You should have a good understanding of the funding source regulations, and your documentation should target areas of occupation that the funding source considers necessary and reimbursable (Hussey et al., 2007; Lohman & Lamb, 2009).

CONTRIBUTING FACTORS

The second part of the problem statement identifies the contributing factors (Table 5-2) that limit engagement in the desired occupation. As described in Chapter 1, the various aspects that comprise occupational therapy's domain are all viewed as having equal value and "together they interact to influence the client's engagement in occupations, participation, and health" (AOTA, 2008b, p. 626). While there may be multiple contributing factors to a limitation in occupational performance, your documentation should focus on those factors that can be addressed through occupational therapy intervention.

Gateley CA, Borcherding S. *Documentation Manual for Occupational Therapy: Writing SOAP Notes, 3rd Edition* (pp. 37-48)
© 2012 SLACK Incorporated

Areas of Occupation

Area of Occupation	Description	Examples
Activities of daily living (ADLs)	Activities necessary for self-care and personal independence. May also be referred to as basic activities of daily living (BADLs) or personal activities of daily living (PADLs)	◆ Bathing/showering ◆ Bowel and bladder management ◆ Dressing ◆ Eating ◆ Feeding ◆ Functional mobility (during performance of functional activities) ◆ Personal device care ◆ Personal hygiene and grooming ◆ Sexual activity ◆ Toilet hygiene
Instrumental activities of daily living (IADLs)	Activities involving participation in the home or community that often require more complex problem-solving and social skills than ADLs	◆ Care of others ◆ Care of pets ◆ Child rearing ◆ Communication management ◆ Community mobility ◆ Financial management ◆ Health management and maintenance ◆ Home establishment and management ◆ Meal preparation and clean up ◆ Religious observance ◆ Safety and emergency maintenance ◆ Shopping
Rest and sleep	Activities related to obtaining the rest and sleep necessary for successful engagement in other areas of occupation	◆ Rest ◆ Sleep ◆ Sleep participation ◆ Sleep preparation
Education	Includes activities necessary for learning and participating in an educational environment	◆ Formal education participation ◆ Informal personal educational needs or interests exploration ◆ Informal personal education participation
Work	Includes seeking and carrying out paid employment or volunteer activities	◆ Employment interests and pursuits ◆ Employment seeking and acquisition ◆ Job performance ◆ Retirement preparation and adjustment ◆ Volunteer exploration ◆ Volunteer participation
Play	Activities that provide enjoyment or entertainment; may be spontaneous or organized	◆ Play exploration ◆ Play participation
Leisure	Intrinsically rewarding activities that are engaged in when an individual is not obligated to perform other occupations	◆ Leisure exploration ◆ Leisure participation
Social participation	Interaction with others that is within expected contextual norms	◆ Community ◆ Family ◆ Peer, friend

Information compiled from American Occupational Therapy Association. (2008). Occupational therapy practice framework: Domain & process, 2nd edition. *American Journal of Occupational Therapy, 62*(6), 625-688.

Table 5-2

Potential Contributing Factors

Potential Contributing Factors	Description	Examples

Client factors	"...specific abilities, characteristics, or beliefs that reside within the client..." (AOTA, 2008b, p. 630)	◆ Values, beliefs, and spirituality
		◆ Body functions
		  • Mental: Attention, memory, perception, sequencing, coping
		  • Sensory: Vision, hearing, vestibular, tactile, pain, proprioceptive
		  • Neuromusculoskeletal: Joint mobility and stability, muscle tone, strength, range of motion, voluntary movement
		  • Cardiovascular, hematological, immunological, and respiratory: Blood pressure, heart rate, physical endurance
		◆ Body structures

Performance skills	"...the abilities that clients demonstrate in the actions they perform." (AOTA, 2008b, p. 640)	◆ Motor and praxis skills: Bending, reaching, pacing, coordinating, maintaining balance, manipulating ◆ Sensory-perceptual skills: Locating, discerning, timing movement ◆ Emotional regulation skills: Controlling anger, responding in an appropriate manner ◆ Cognitive skills: Judging, sequencing, organizing, prioritizing, multitasking ◆ Communication and social skills: Looking, gesturing, taking turns
Performance patterns	Patterns of behavior related to the activities of an individual, organization, or population	◆ Habits: Repetitive rocking in response to stress ◆ Routines: Morning routine for dressing and grooming; follows chain of command at workplace ◆ Rituals: Holiday meal preparation ◆ Roles: Caregiver, worker, student

Context and environment	"...a variety of interrelated conditions within and surrounding the client..." (AOTA, 2008b, p. 645)	◆ Cultural: Customs, beliefs, ethnicity, politics
		◆ Personal: Age, gender, socioeconomic status, educational status
		◆ Temporal: Stage of life, time of day, time of year, duration, history
		◆ Virtual: Communication via airway or computer
		◆ Physical:
		  • Natural environment: Terrain, plants and animals, sensory qualities
		  • Built environment: Buildings, objects, tools, devices
		◆ Social: Presence, relationships and expectations of others

Activity demands	"...the specific features of an activity that influence the type and amount of effort required to perform an activity." (AOTA, 2008b, p. 634)	◆ Objects and properties: Tools, materials, equipment ◆ Space demands: Physical environmental requirements ◆ Social demands: Rules, expectations ◆ Sequence and timing: Processes, steps ◆ Required actions and performance skills: Skills necessary to carry out the activity ◆ Required body functions: Joint mobility, sustained attention ◆ Required body structures: Both hands, both eyes

Information compiled from American Occupational Therapy Association. (2008). Occupational therapy practice framework: Domain & process, 2nd edition. *American Journal of Occupational Therapy, 62*(6), 625-688.

WRITING PROBLEM STATEMENTS

> Note: In this manual, the terms *client, patient, student, child, infant, consumer, resident, individual, veteran,* and first names have been used to reflect the terms used in various practice settings. Names have been fabricated to protect the confidentiality of those people who receive our services. If a note says, "Mr. P was seen in his home…" please understand that he is being called "Mr. P" for purposes of confidentiality. In your documentation, please use the term or format that is considered most respectful in your setting.

As occupational therapy practitioners, we recognize that a client's sense of well-being depends partly on the ability to participate in the life roles desired at home, at work, at school, and in the community. Through various evaluation procedures, we identify the areas of occupation impacted by a client's condition and the factors contributing to the functional limitation. Whenever possible, we also specify the extent to which occupational performance is limited. It is important to note that *the client's diagnosis is not the problem.* The contributing factors may be the result of the diagnosis, but it is our responsibility to identify those specific factors that contribute to functional limitation. To summarize, you need to identify the following:

✦ An area of occupation
  • If possible, a measurement of the functional limitation
✦ A contributing factor to be addressed in occupational therapy
  • If possible, a measurement for the contributing factor
  • Optional: The diagnosis causing this factor

Let's take a look at an example of a functional problem statement:

Client is <u>unable to dress self</u> Ⓘ due to ↓ <u>AROM in Ⓑ UE</u>.
       Area of Occupation   Contributing Factor

This statement has the essential elements of the area of occupation and a contributing factor, but more specific measurable information would be helpful in documenting progress toward goals. Based on the problem statement above, you will not be able to show any increase in function until the client demonstrates full active range of motion (AROM) and is independent in dressing. Rather than saying that the client is **unable to perform** a given activity independently, it is better to state the assist level needed. It is also helpful to provide the **amount** of AROM that is limited.

For example:
Client requires max Ⓐ to dress self due to ½ AROM in Ⓑ UE.

With this reworded problem statement, you now will be able to document progress when the client demonstrates an increase in AROM or when the client is able to complete dressing with mod Ⓐ. It may also be helpful to add the diagnosis.

For example:
Client requires max Ⓐ to dress self due to ½ AROM in Ⓑ UE 2° to infection of the spinal cord.

It is not mandatory to list the diagnosis in the problem statement since it will be documented in other parts of your initial evaluation. In some cases, however, it is helpful to document the diagnosis since there may be a difference in the interventions that will be provided based on the diagnosis.

> For ease of writing, you can use the following formula to write a functional problem statement:
>
> Client requires _____ in _____ due to _____.
>   assist level   performing what occupational task   contributing factor

A few more examples:
✦ *Child requires mod Ⓐ to hold scissors to complete art activities in school due to high tone in Ⓡ UE.*
✦ *Veteran requires min Ⓐ in completing toilet transfer due to trunk instability resulting from Ⓡ CVA.*
✦ *Consumer requires maximal verbal cues to complete 3-step lunch preparation due to decreased sequencing and problem-solving skills.*

If a client is unable to perform an activity independently, the assist level will be specified. However, sometimes the activity is one that the client either **can** or **cannot** do, with no assist levels in question. In that case, you can use the following format:

Client unable to _____ due to _____.
　　　　　　　　　　engage in what occupational task　　　　　　　　　　what contributing factor

For example:

✦ *Consumer is unable to sustain employment more than 2 weeks due to absence of stress management skills.*

✦ *Client is unable to grasp a writing instrument for more than 3 minutes due to pain level of >5/10 with finger flexion of Ⓡ hand.*

✦ *Child is unable to do jumping jacks to participate in gym class due to motor planning deficits.*

In the last example, the child cannot do the task with any level of assistance. It is a "can" or "cannot" activity. The child is not dependent in jumping jacks; she just cannot do them.

It is not mandatory that the formats above be used. These are useful ways of wording functional problem statements, but there are others. Sometimes a slightly different format is more useful:

_____ results in _____.
　　　　　Contributing factor　　　　　　　　　　　　　what occupational deficit

For example:

✦ *Three steps leading to front door limit client's independence in entering house.*

✦ *Inability to perform simple math calculations results in need for caregiver assistance in IADL tasks such as balancing checkbook.*

✦ *Pain level >6 at end range shoulder flexion limits ability to don shirt overhead.*

✦ *Aggressive behavior results in limited opportunities for social participation and repeated involvement with the juvenile justice system.*

EXAMPLES OF FUNCTIONAL PROBLEM STATEMENTS

When formulating problem statements, be sure the problem identified is one that will respond to occupational therapy treatment. There is no need to identify problems that you do not intend to treat. As previously stated, you also need to focus on problems for which treatment is considered necessary and reimbursable by the funding source.

Note: There is a cardstock pullout at the end of this manual that lists the three formulas for writing functional problem statements as well as several examples. Pull it out and carry it with you to use as a quick reference guide.

ACTIVITIES OF DAILY LIVING

✦ *Individual requires verbal and tactile cues 100% of time in order to stay on task, initiate, and sequence during dressing activity.*

✦ *Client requires mod Ⓐ to don pants 2° 3+ UE strength.*

✦ *Patient requires mod verbal cues and mod physical assist with upper body dressing 2° attention span of <5 minutes.*

✦ *Client tolerates less than 10 minutes of ADL participation due to severe shortness of breath.*

✦ *Veteran requires max Ⓐ in combing hair with Ⓡ UE due to 5 out of 10 Ⓡ elbow pain.*

✦ *Resident requires hand over hand assist to keep food on fork due to poor motor planning.*

✦ *Oral tactile defensiveness results in limited variety of food intake.*

✦ *Patient requires min Ⓐ in dressing activities 2° low vision.*

✦ *Client requires mod Ⓐ for safe bathing 2° poor balance and lack of adaptive equipment.*

+ *Child needs mod Ⓐ in upper body hygiene 2° pronator spasticity which limits Ⓡ forearm supination by ½ range.*
+ *Resident needs max Ⓐ for bed mobility in preparation for dressing secondary to decreased strength in trunk and UEs.*
+ *Child unable to feed self due to asymmetrical positioning in w/c.*
+ *Client is dependent on caregiver to empty catheter bag due to limited Ⓑ UE function resulting from C5 SCI.*

INSTRUMENTAL ACTIVITIES OF DAILY LIVING

+ *Impaired short-term memory results in safety concerns during meal preparation and child care.*
+ *Client unsafe in home management tasks secondary to inability to recognize fatigue when standing.*
+ *Client demonstrates ↓ safety in all IADL tasks due to impaired judgment and sequencing.*
+ *Focused attention on auditory hallucinations makes consumer unsafe to live alone.*
+ *Client requires mod verbal cues for safety during cooking tasks due to impaired Ⓡ UE sensation.*
+ *Client unable to complete laundry tasks due to lifting restrictions in post-surgical back precautions.*
+ *Client unable to write checks for bill paying due to limited grip strength and coordination of dominant Ⓡ hand.*
+ *Resident unable to locate emergency fire exit due to decreased memory and problem solving.*
+ *Frequent alcohol use impairs consumer's ability to operate a motor vehicle safely.*
+ *Client requires max verbal cues to navigate city bus route to doctor's office due to impaired sequencing and problem solving.*
+ *Inability to count money limits client's ability to make independent purchases in the community.*
+ *Client is unable to change infant's diaper due to decreased strength and sensation in Ⓑ hands.*

REST AND SLEEP

+ *Auditory hallucinations result in client obtaining <3 hours sleep nightly.*
+ *Impaired judgment results in resident not calling for assistance when needing to use commode during the night.*
+ *Client requires mod Ⓐ to manage bed linens in preparation for sleep due to impaired sensation and strength of Ⓑ hands resulting from multiple sclerosis.*

EDUCATION

+ *Sierra requires mod Ⓐ to complete art assignment requiring use of a ruler 2° bilateral incoordination.*
+ *Xavier requires step-by-step verbal cues to obtain lunch tray and pay attendant due to impaired sequencing and problem solving.*
+ *Sensory-seeking behaviors and decreased attention result in inability to complete classroom assignments in a timely manner.*
+ *Slow handwriting speed related to Juvenile Rheumatoid Arthritis results in client's inability to keep up with note-taking during college lectures.*

WORK

+ *Preference for youth-culture specific dress limits client's ability to find employment.*
+ *Inattention to personal hygiene interferes with consumer's ability to find employment.*
+ *Client is unable to perform carpentry work due to grip strength of 3# in Ⓡ hand.*
+ *Patient unable to grasp and hold tool with Ⓛ hand due to pain level >5/10 with flexion of Ⓛ index finger.*
+ *<60° AROM in Ⓡ shoulder abduction limits client's ability to perform work tasks.*
+ *Daily cocaine use results in client's inability to hold a job.*
+ *Client requires assistance to complete electronic job application due to decreased vision.*
+ *Client unable to complete volunteer duties at hospital gift shop due to decreased endurance.*
+ *Client unable to lift and carry 20# bucket to feed farm animals due to decreased balance.*

Play

+ *Preoccupation with aligning objects limits child's pretend play interactions with preschool classmates.*
+ *Child needs max verbal and tactile cues to transfer toys from one hand to the other due to inattention to Ⓡ side of the body.*
+ *Elisio is unable to engage in age-appropriate play activities due to sensory processing deficits.*
+ *Adolescent requires mod verbal cues for turn taking during group board games due to impulsive behaviors.*

Leisure

+ *Resident unable to complete needlework due to impaired coordination of Ⓡ hand.*
+ *Impaired problem-solving skills limit consumer's ability to utilize public transportation to attend weekly bowling league.*
+ *Client requires mod Ⓐ to manage camera functions when taking pictures.*

Social Participation

+ *Belief in government conspiracy limits consumer's willingness to participate socially.*
+ *Child unable to communicate with peers verbally due to progressive oral motor weakness resulting from muscular dystrophy.*
+ *Anxiety in crowds limits client's willingness to leave home for participation in social events.*
+ *Individual's aggressive behavior results in social isolation.*
+ *Drug-seeking and drug-using behaviors limit client's social participation in non–drug-related activities.*

WORKSHEET 5-1

Identifying the Contributing Factors

Complete each of the following functional problem statements with at least three possible contributing factors. (Hint: It may be helpful to refer to Table 5-2 for potential contributing factors.)

1. *Area of Occupation = Work*

   • Consumer is unable to sustain employment longer than 2 weeks due to

   • Consumer is unable to sustain employment longer than 2 weeks due to

   • Consumer is unable to sustain employment longer than 2 weeks due to

2. *Area of Occupation = ADLs*

   • Veteran needs 1 ½ hours to complete grooming tasks due to

   • Veteran needs 1 ½ hours to complete grooming tasks due to

   • Veteran needs 1 ½ hours to complete grooming tasks due to

3. *Area of Occupation = Education*

   • Child is unable to complete grade-appropriate written worksheets due to

   • Child is unable to complete grade-appropriate written worksheets due to

   • Child is unable to complete grade-appropriate written worksheets due to

WORKSHEET 5-2

Writing Functional Problem Statements

Use the following descriptions to write functional problem statements for each client. Make them specific enough to:

✦ Show the area of occupation that is a concern
✦ Show the contributing factor(s) that impact this area of occupation
✦ Serve as a baseline against which to measure progress

You may use any of the three formats provided in this chapter for writing the functional problem statements.

1. *The client has an acquired injury to his brain. As a result, he is not able to pay attention to task for very long at a time, and he is having trouble completing his morning routine. Usually he can pay attention to what he is doing for about 2 minutes, and needs to be redirected back to the task after that.*

2. *The child is having trouble in school because she has difficulty staying within the lines when she is writing. She habitually grips her pencil in a gross grasp, although with help (someone's hand placed over hers) she can hold it with her thumb and two fingers.*

3. *The resident is not very cognitively aware. About 40% of the time she has trouble figuring out what to do first if she has to complete a self-care task, and she doesn't remember what she has just been told.*

4. *Mr. J has recently sustained a Ⓡ CVA. His Ⓛ arm is flaccid and he forgets that it is there. He needs physical and verbal help with ADL tasks about 60% of the time.*

5. *The consumer has had trouble finding a job. His appearance is unkempt and he has a strong body odor, neither of which seem troubling to him.*

6. *The client is unable to transfer safely w/c ↔ toilet without someone to remind him that he needs to follow his total hip precautions.*

Writing Measurable Occupation-Based Goals and Objectives

Goals and objectives used in a treatment plan must be written in occupation-based, measurable, observable, action-oriented terms. They must also be realistic for the client and able to be achieved in a reasonable amount of time. Goals are formulated from the problem list you have compiled in collaboration with the client. For successful intervention, it is critical that you work on goals that are important to the client. "Occupational therapy practitioners have an ethical responsibility to include clients in discussions regarding their own care and to provide them with the opportunity to share in the decisions that affect them" (Rosa, 2009, p. 289).

Occupational therapy goals must focus on functional improvements in occupational performance. The client factors that contribute to such progress, such as strength and range of motion, are much less important to a third-party payer than what the client can actually do, even though the gains in those contributing factors may be essential to achieving the functional outcome.

As a profession, we are increasingly being asked to demonstrate that our services are necessary and cost-effective (Lohman & Lamb, 2009). There is also a movement toward evidence-based practice and communicating that evidence in clinical documentation (Davis, Zayat, Urton, Belgum, & Hill, 2008). Tickle-Degnen (2009) suggests that occupational therapy practitioners combine scientific research evidence with the information that is gathered through interviews and observations of clients. Using this approach, we can collaborate with our clients to establish outcome measures that demonstrate functional improvements and the ability to participate in meaningful occupation.

GOALS

Goals in an intervention plan are also called *long-term goals* (LTG) or outcomes. These are usually discharge goals—what the client hopes to accomplish by the time of discharge from occupational therapy services. For each problem you have identified, you will have at least one LTG, and often more than one.

OBJECTIVES

Objectives are also called *short-term goals* (STG). These are goals that are met in daily or weekly increments while progressing toward the discharge goals.

For example, if your LTG is:
   Client will complete 3-step stove top meal preparation with modified independence using walker by 7/15/11.

then one of your STGs might be:
   Client will retrieve and transport items from refrigerator to stove using walker and wheeled cart with CGA by 7/5/11.

Gateley CA, Borcherding S. *Documentation Manual for Occupational Therapy: Writing SOAP Notes, 3rd Edition* (pp. 49-62)
© 2012 SLACK Incorporated

If your LTG is:

Client will move 35# objects needed for work from table to counter without ↑ in pain by 12/18/11.

then one of your STGs might be:

Client will be able to lift 10# objects needed for work without ↑ in pain by 12/5/11.

You may have several STGs (objectives) for each LTG. For example, suppose you are treating Mr. Hawkins, a 45-year-old executive who sustained a ⓡ CVA a few days ago and has ⓛ hemiplegia. On evaluation, you find that he is oriented X 4, verbal, intelligent, able to learn, and has a supportive wife. After talking with him about what he would like to achieve in occupational therapy, you and he decide upon a goal of independent upper body dressing. You believe that this is a realistic goal, provided that he receives skilled instruction and the necessary adaptive equipment. You set a series of STGs:

1. Seated edge of bed, client will reach for clothing items at arm's length with CGA to maintain dynamic sitting by the end of the 3rd treatment session.

2. By the 6th treatment session, client will be able to tolerate >10 minutes of dressing activity without rest break seated edge of bed with CGA.

3. After skilled instruction, client will be able to don shirt sitting EOB using one-handed techniques with min verbal cues by 7/10/11.

4. Client will be able to button shirt using a button hook with 2 or fewer verbal cues by 7/12/11.

5. Client will complete all upper body dressing tasks with modified independence seated EOB by 7/15/11.

As you can see, each of these STGs is measurable, observable, and action-oriented. The first four STGs are steps to the ultimate LTG (Figure 6-1).

Figure 6-1. Steps to the ultimate LTG.

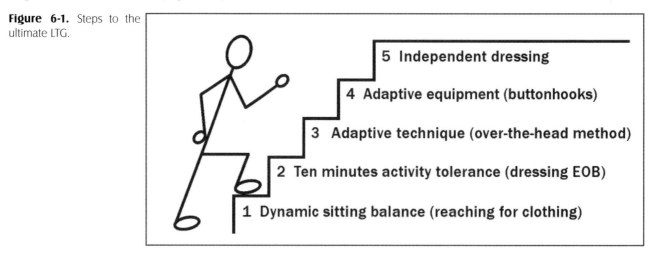

5 **Independent dressing**

4 **Adaptive equipment (buttonhooks)**

3 **Adaptive technique (over-the-head method)**

2 **Ten minutes activity tolerance (dressing EOB)**

1 **Dynamic sitting balance (reaching for clothing)**

An intervention plan is always a work in progress. Unexpected events and conditions can impact the progress your client will be able to make toward his or her goals. If you find a goal unrealistic, you are obligated to change it. It is not useful to continue with a plan that is not working. For example, suppose that your client begins to have some motor return in his involved ⓛ upper extremity. You now know that he may be able to dress his upper body without adaptive techniques or equipment, and he wants very much to do that. You would need to write a new set of STGs for him.

GOAL WRITING: THE COAST METHOD

There are several formats available for writing goal statements (Sames, 2010). In this manual, we will present a new format: the COAST method. This method was designed around the principles put forth by Crepeau et al. (2009a) that contemporary practice should be client-centered and occupation-centered. Just as the SOAP format is one way of learning to document occupational therapy services, the COAST method is simply one way of learning to write goals. While settings may vary in the format used, learning the COAST method will ensure that you consistently include all necessary information in your goal statements.

- ✦ C–Client   Client will perform
- ✦ O–Occupation   What occupation?
- ✦ A–Assist Level   With what level of assistance/independence?
- ✦ S–Specific Condition   Under what conditions?
- ✦ T–Timeline   By when?

There has been considerable debate about the concepts of *occupation*, *activity*, and *task*, with definitions varying between conceptual models (Brown, 2009). It is not within the scope of this textbook to engage in that debate. The *Framework-II* (AOTA, 2008b) provides multiple definitions of occupation that include the terms *activity* or *task*. For purposes of this textbook, it can be assumed that the "O" in the COAST acronym encompasses any activity or task that is related to the performance of an area of occupation as defined by the *Framework-II* (AOTA, 2008b).

In order to write goals and objectives in a way that can be measured, the elements to be included are very specific. Let's take a closer look at each category.

C (CLIENT)

In writing treatment goals, the **client** is the key player. Goals should be written in terms of what the client will do, <u>not what the therapist will do</u>. The therapist's actions are documented later, under intervention strategies. An action verb is also inserted here, such as *perform*, *demonstrate*, or *complete*.

For example:
> *Client will perform*...

O (OCCUPATION)

This is the specific **occupation** to which this goal pertains and should relate to the problem statements that have been established. Improving an individual's ability to engage in occupation is the core of occupational therapy practice. It is the first thing you think of in writing goals, and it should be the essential focus of the goal statement.

For example:
> *Client will perform <u>a 3-step cooking process</u>*...

A (ASSIST LEVEL)

This is where you specify the level of assistance expected, which ultimately translates into the level of independence that the client is expected to demonstrate. This should include the physical and/or verbal cues that will be required in order for the client to complete the activity.

For example:
> *Client will perform a 3-step cooking process <u>with 2 or fewer verbal cues for sequencing and safety</u>*...

Note: The method used to describe the level of assistance will vary between settings and funding sources. For example, settings in which Medicare is a primary funding source, such as inpatient rehabilitation centers and long-term care facilities, often use the Functional Independence Measure (FIM) instrument as a common measure of client outcomes (UDSMR, 2010). You need to be aware of the common terminology used in your setting and incorporate it into your goal writing.

S (SPECIFIC CONDITIONS)

This is where you specify any other conditions under which the client is expected to perform the desired action such as location, adaptive equipment, or modified technique.

For example:
> *Client will perform a 3-step cooking process with 2 or fewer verbal cues for sequencing and safety <u>from w/c level in rehab kitchen</u>*...

The "A" and "S" together make your goal statement **measurable** and allow you to show your client's progress. Other examples include:

✦ *...by using a dressing stick with 2 or fewer verbal cues*

✦ *...using walker with CGA*

✦ *...with mod Ⓐ using sliding board*

✦ *...3 out of 4 attempts without verbal cues*

✦ *...independently from standing position*

✦ *...using medication organizer with weekly supervision for set-up*

✦ *...3 out of 5 attempts during evening meal*

✦ *...with modified independence using tub bench and hand-held shower hose*

✦ *...during group sessions without use of profanity*

In some cases, it is acceptable to omit either the "A" or the "S," **but never both**. You may write a goal for a task that either can or cannot be done, and assistance would not be applicable. For example, suppose you have a client who presents with pain in her Ⓡ CMC joint. She is able to complete most IADL tasks independently, but reports pain during tasks such as opening doorknobs. Your LTG may look like this:

Client will open doorknobs using Ⓡ hand without report of wrist pain within 2 weeks.

In this example, no assist level is mentioned but "without report of wrist pain" makes this goal measurable.

Another example:

Client will complete all dressing tasks Ⓘ by 7/21/2011.

In this example, the assistance level (or in this case the lack of assistance level) is stated, but there are no other specific conditions that are necessary for this goal.

T (Timeline)

This is the timeframe within which the goal is expected to be accomplished. For a **LTG**, this may be the anticipated discharge date.

For example:

✦ *Client will perform a 3-step cooking process with 2 or fewer verbal cues for sequencing and safety from w/c level in rehab kitchen <u>by 3/20/11</u>.*

✦ *Client will perform a 3-step cooking process with 2 or fewer verbal cues for sequencing and safety from w/c level in rehab kitchen <u>within 2 weeks</u>.*

Depending on your setting, the timeline for your **STGs** may be daily, weekly, or by number of sessions.

For example:

✦ *Client will prepare a sandwich with 2 or fewer verbal cues for sequencing and safety from w/c level in rehab kitchen <u>by 3/16/11</u>.*

✦ *Client will prepare a sandwich with 2 or fewer verbal cues for sequencing and safety from w/c level in rehab kitchen <u>within 1 week</u>.*

✦ *Client will prepare a sandwich with 2 or fewer verbal cues for sequencing and safety from w/c level in rehab kitchen <u>by 5th treatment session</u>.*

EXAMPLES OF GOAL STATEMENTS

The COAST method is useful as you are learning to write, although the order may need to be changed slightly in order for your sentence to make sense. **As long as all of the required elements are present, it does not matter with which element you begin your sentence.** Let's take a look at a few examples:

C: *Client will*

O: *feed self 50% of meal*

A: *with min physical Ⓐ to scoop*

S: *using built-up spoon*

T: *within 3 tx. sessions.*

The elements of this goal statement can be rearranged without changing the meaning of the goal:

✦ *Within 3 tx. sessions, client will feed self 50% of meal using built-up spoon with min physical Ⓐ to scoop.*

✦ *Using built-up spoon, client will feed self 50% of meal with min physical Ⓐ to scoop within 3 sessions.*

Here is another example:

C:	*Client will perform*
O:	*bed-making activity*
A:	*with min verbal cues*
S:	*while adhering to postsurgical back precautions*
T:	*by 12/12/11.*

The elements of this goal statement can be rearranged without changing the meaning of the goal:

With min verbal cues, client will perform bed-making activity while adhering to postsurgical back precautions by 12/11/11.

ACTIVITIES OF DAILY LIVING

✦ *Brittney will don coat using over-the-head method Ⓘ within 1 month.*

✦ *Client will fasten 3 buttons in 2 minutes using button hook with min verbal cues by 5/2/11.*

✦ *Within 3 treatment sessions, Mr. S will complete toileting using raised toilet seat with min Ⓐ for balance during clothing adjustment.*

✦ *Pt. will complete bathing tasks seated on tub bench using long-handled sponge with SBA within 1 week.*

✦ *Child will feed self 50% of meal using adaptive spoon with mod Ⓐ within 3 weeks.*

✦ *Pt. will empty catheter leg-bag with min verbal cues for technique within 1 week.*

✦ *Client will demonstrate safe clothing retrieval and transport from closet using walker with CGA by 11/30/11.*

✦ *Caregiver will demonstrate correct application of client's postsurgical back corset during upper body dressing tasks without verbal cues by end of 2nd treatment session.*

INSTRUMENTAL ACTIVITIES OF DAILY LIVING

✦ *Client will transfer 10 laundry items from washer to dryer with 3 or fewer verbal cues to adhere to postsurgical back precautions by 6/23/2011.*

✦ *Client will demonstrate ability to change infant's diaper using adaptive one-handed methods with 2 or fewer verbal cues within 2 weeks.*

✦ *Client will analyze bill statement and write check for correct amount 3 of 4 attempts with min verbal cues by 8/19/11.*

✦ *Within 3 days, client will demonstrate safe transfer in/out of car with supervision while adhering to postsurgical hip precautions.*

✦ *Resident will identify and navigate safe route from bedroom to exit of residential care facility independently by 7/5/11.*

✦ *Client will locate phone numbers of emergency services in the telephone directory without physical or verbal cues by end of 3rd treatment session.*

✦ *Ryan will navigate public bus system from home to doctor's office with supervision during next treatment session.*

REST AND SLEEP

✦ *Using visual checklist as memory aid, client will remember to lock doors before bedtime on 5 consecutive nights by 9/21/11.*

✦ *Consumer will go to bed before midnight at least 75% of weeknights within 2 weeks in order to obtain adequate sleep for effective participation at job.*

EDUCATION

Note: Therapists working in public schools use a slightly different terminology. In education, goals for one school year are called **objectives** or **behavioral objectives**. Educational goals often are not measured by time, such as *by 5/7/11* or *within 3 weeks*. Since the Individualized Education Program (IEP) is written annually, the time frame for educational goals is assumed to be annual. Children sometimes exhibit a new behavior inconsistently before it is really established. Therefore, measurement used for children is more likely to reflect whether the behavior is <u>established</u>. For example:

Min Jung will obtain and transport lunch tray to table Ⓘ from w/c level 9 of 10 days.

- *Taneisha independently will cut out circle during classroom activities using supinated grasp on scissors with <2 deviations 75% of attempts.*
- *Child will maintain seated position at desk for 5 minutes with 2 or fewer verbal cues 4/5 attempts.*
- *Child independently will print upper case alphabet on wide-ruled notebook paper, demonstrating proper letter formation and staying on line, with <3 errors 75% of attempts.*
- *Student will don/doff coat without physical assistance 90% of the time in order to be independent with beginning and end-of-day school routine.*
- *Isabella will take turns on playground equipment without adult intervention 3 of 4 consecutive days.*
- *Child will copy 10 math problems from whiteboard to paper with <2 errors and no verbal cues 80% of attempts.*
- *Ethan will complete assigned classroom tasks within allotted time with fewer than 3 verbal cues 75% of the time.*
- *Lily will participate in group activities for up to 10 minutes without exhibiting aggressive behaviors toward classmates 4 of 5 consecutive days.*

WORK

- *Jervon independently will request at least one job application from a restaurant within 1 week.*
- *Client will transfer 10# boxes from floor to shelf during simulated work tasks, demonstrating proper body mechanics without verbal cues by 10/17/2011.*
- *By 5/4/11, client will count correct change from a $20 bill without verbal cues in order to return to position as volunteer in hospital gift shop.*
- *Carlos independently will identify at least 2 opportunities for community volunteer service by next group session.*
- *Client will navigate power w/c in work environment without bumping into objects or people within 3 weeks.*
- *Client will demonstrate ability to type 20 words per minute during simulated work tasks using Ⓑ wrist cock-up splints within 2 weeks.*

PLAY

- *Infant will visually track a toy 45 degrees past midline in both directions during play activities on 3 of 4 attempts by 6/30/11.*
- *DeShawn will use Ⓛ UE as a functional assist 5/5 opportunities during spontaneous play within 2 months.*
- *Child will place 3 shapes into puzzle board with no verbal cues in 3 months.*
- *Katrina will engage in pretend play activity with peers for >3 minutes with minimal adult facilitation by 2/28/12.*
- *Infant will engage in Ⓑ UE play activity while independently sitting unsupported >1 minute by 10/10/11.*
- *Child will catch tennis ball in Ⓑ hands on 8 of 10 attempts when tossed from 10 feet within 3 weeks.*
- *Lauren independently will stack 6 or more 1" blocks using Ⓡ hand to stabilize tower within 1 month.*

SOCIAL PARTICIPATION

✦ *Consumer independently will choose and participate in at least one social activity per week 3/3 weeks within 1 month.*

✦ *With mod verbal cues, consumer will ask roommate to smoke outside the building next time the situation arises.*

✦ *Deondré will make at least 2 verbal contributions to group discussions with min verbal prompts 5/5 days within 2 weeks.*

✦ *Child will tolerate unexpected touch from peers during circle time without demonstrating aggressive behaviors 80% of the time per daycare provider report.*

✦ *Using visual schedule and min verbal cues, child will transition between home and preschool environment without expressing anxiety or fear at least 50% of the time within 3 months.*

LEISURE

✦ *Client independently will identify at least 3 leisure activities that are not associated with drinking by 9/8/11.*

✦ *Within 3 weeks, client will demonstrate sufficient coordination to manipulate toothpaste caps, buttons, and knitting needles without dropping.*

> Note: There is a cardstock pullout at the end of this manual that reviews the COAST formula and provides several examples of goal statements. Pull it out and carry it with you to use as a quick-reference guide.

Medical Necessity

As occupational therapists, we view a client holistically, considering the whole person with his or her needs, interests, problems, strengths, and priorities. We know that leisure is an important part of the total picture. When this is the client's priority, we might be inclined to write problem statements and goals focusing on leisure skills and interests, such as:

✦ Problem: *Client is unable to play softball due to ↓ AROM and ↑ pain in ℝ wrist.*

✦ LTG: *Client will pitch a softball without wrist pain within 6 weeks.*

However, we know that both Medicare and private insurance are very frugal with our health care dollars and approve expenditures only for medical necessity. Since even adaptive equipment such as a raised toilet seat is not always considered medically necessary, treatment focused on a client's leisure goals is likely to be denied under our current reimbursement system. In consideration of the client's holistic needs and the reimbursement limitations, instead we may address in the intervention plan some of the contributing factors that enable the client to perform a variety of functional tasks. Documentation would focus on goals and interventions that provide the client with skills for self-care and work, as well as the leisure activities so important to the quality of life. Worksheet 6-1 will allow you to practice this documentation skill.

In the example above, we might suspect that the client is also having difficulty with household or work tasks requiring ℝ UE use. It would be more appropriate to write an IADL goal, such as:

Client will lift pots and pans during dishwashing without wrist pain in 6 weeks.

Interventions would be targeted toward the client factors of AROM and pain, and improvements in these client factors would result in an increased ability for the client to pursue her leisure interests as well.

> Note: **DO NOT** use participation in treatment as a goal. For example:
>
> *Client will do 20 reps of shoulder ladder with 1# wt. in order to ↑ endurance to become more ① in IADLs.*
>
> Instead, write a goal that specifies the amount of endurance the client needs to demonstrate during an occupation-based activity. For example:
>
> *Client will complete seated cooking task >5 minutes without rest breaks with SBA within 2 weeks.*

Goals in Different Settings

The COAST format works well in many occupational therapy settings. This method of goal writing allows you to demonstrate the specific need for occupational therapy services by focusing on areas of occupation impacted by the client's condition. In some settings, problem statements and goals are written differently due to the nature of services provided.

Mental Health and Substance Abuse

In mental health and substance abuse practice settings, problem statements and goals are often multidisciplinary and are written to be addressed by the treatment team rather than by one specific discipline.

For example:
+ Problem: *Alcohol use*
+ Behavioral manifestation: *Kyle admits to drinking 8 oz. of liquor and 7 to 8 beers nightly, resulting in failing grades and involvement with the law due to fighting with fists and weapons.*
+ Short-term goal: *By next group session, Kyle will identify 2 leisure activities not associated with drinking.*

Another example:
+ Problem: *Noncompliant behavior*
+ Behavioral manifestation: *Bianca is noncompliant with family rules and social norms (attending school, abiding by the law), resulting in assignment to a parole officer and 3 failed foster home placements.*
+ Short-term goal: *Bianca will demonstrate willingness to cooperate with family norms by entering into a behavioral contract with her parents within 1 week.*

Early Intervention

In recent years, early intervention programs that provide services for children age birth to 3 years have moved toward a family-centered, transdisciplinary model of service delivery (Myers et al., 2010). One aspect of a family-centered approach is that rather than the professionals setting the goals for the child, families identify the "outcomes" that they hope their child will achieve. For example, the family may identify outcomes such as the following:

+ *Logan will use words during playtime and meals to express his needs.*
+ *Logan will express his emotion in positive ways when he is excited.*
+ *Logan will show interest in potty training.*
+ *Logan will walk up and down the stairs at home unassisted.*
+ *Logan will use a spoon to feed himself at least half of his meal.*

The transdisciplinary aspect of early intervention means that families will interact directly with only one or two individuals of the team on a regular basis, with other disciplines providing services on a consultative basis. Occupational therapists providing early intervention services under a transdisciplinary model may encounter the need for role release, which is "the commitment of professionals to teaching, learning, and providing direct services that may not be traditionally within their discipline-specific roles" (Mulligan, 2003, pp. 240-241). If you work in an early intervention setting, your documentation and interventions should reflect the service delivery model required by the agency.

WORKSHEET 6-1

Choosing Goals for Medical Necessity

Below is a scenario for a client who has stated a priority for leisure interests. You will have the opportunity to write goals that focus on other areas of occupation while still addressing the same contributing factors that are impacting her performance of leisure activities.

- ✦ Problem: *Client unable to perform sewing due to 2+/5 strength in Ⓡ hand musculature.*
  - • LTG: *Client will perform embroidery Ⓘ for 20 minutes within 8 weeks.*
  - • STG: *In order to ↑ performance of embroidery, client will use needle continuously for 5 minutes within 2 weeks.*

1. What other problems might this woman have due to decreased strength in her Ⓡ hand?

2. What long-term goal might you use that would show medical necessity for increasing Ⓡ UE strength?

3. What short-term goal might be used as a step to achieve that LTG?

WORKSHEET 6-2

Evaluating Goal Statements

Refer to the COAST elements to determine which of the following goals has each of the necessary components to be useful in occupational therapy documentation. For each goal that you find to be incomplete or inaccurate in some way, indicate what is missing.

1. *By the time of discharge in 2 weeks, client will dress himself with min Ⓐ for balance using a sock aid and reacher while sitting in w/c.*
   ___ This goal has all of the necessary COAST components.
   ___ This goal lacks:

2. *Client will tolerate 10 minutes of treatment daily.*
   ___ This goal has all of the necessary COAST components.
   ___ This goal lacks:

3. *Client will demonstrate increased coping skills when communicating with her daughter within 2 weeks.*
   ___ This goal has all of the necessary COAST components.
   ___ This goal lacks:

4. *Client will demonstrate 15 minutes of activity tolerance without rest breaks using Ⓑ UEs in order to complete ADL tasks before breakfast each morning.*
   ___ This goal has all of the necessary COAST components.
   ___ This goal lacks:

5. *OT will teach lower body dressing using a reacher, dressing stick, and sock aide within 3 treatment sessions.*
   ___ This goal has all of the necessary COAST components.
   ___ This goal lacks:

6. *Patient will demonstrate ability to balance his checkbook.*
   ___ This goal has all of the necessary COAST components.
   ___ This goal lacks:

WORKSHEET 6-3

Writing Client-Centered, Occupation-Based, Measurable Goals

Write goals for the scenarios below that are client-centered, occupation-based, and measureable. Please remember that we set goals <u>with</u> the client. Assume for this worksheet that you have already collaborated with the client regarding his or her goals.

1. Shontelle is not able to attend to task for more than a few minutes, which makes IADL activities difficult for her. Since she likes to cook and plans to return to cooking after discharge, you have been working with her in the kitchen. You would like to see her able to attend to task for 10 minutes by the time she is discharged next week. Write a goal that addresses Shontelle's attention span during cooking.

    C: _____
        (Client will perform)

    O: _____
        (Occupation)

    A: _____
        (Assist level)

    S: _____
        (Specific conditions)

    T: _____
        (Timeline—by when?)

2. Now write a goal for Shontelle to be able to follow directions so that she can read the back of a boxed meal, and eventually a recipe, when she is cooking.

    C: _____
        (Client will perform)

    O: _____
        (Occupation)

    A: _____
        (Assist level)

    S: _____
        (Specific conditions)

    T: _____
        (Timeline—by when?)

3. Bill is having trouble dressing himself after his stroke. You have been teaching him an over-the-head method for putting on his shirt, and have given him a buttonhook to use. Write a dressing goal for Bill.

    C: _____
        (Client will perform)

    O: _____
        (Occupation)

    A: _____
        (Assist level)

    S: _____
        (Specific conditions)

    T: _____
        (Timeline—by when?)

WORKSHEET 6-3 (CONTINUED)

Writing Client-Centered, Occupation-Based, Measurable Goals

Write goals for the scenarios below that are client-centered, occupation-based, and measureable. Please remember that we set goals <u>with</u> the client. Assume for this worksheet that you have already collaborated with the client regarding his or her goals.

4. Abigail is very weak, and she wants to be able to go back to work as a receptionist. She also wants to be able to care for her 4-month-old child. Write a goal that addresses her activity tolerance during an occupation-based activity.

   C: _____
      (Client will perform)

   O: _____
      (Occupation)

   A: _____
      (Assist level)

   S: _____
      (Specific conditions)

   T: _____
      (Timeline—by when?)

5. Rashad wants to live independently in the community, but lacks basic money management skills. Write a goal for Rashad to improve his money management skills.

   C: _____
      (Client will perform)

   O: _____
      (Occupation)

   A: _____
      (Assist level)

   S: _____
      (Specific conditions)

   T: _____
      (Timeline—by when?)

6. Kylie has become increasingly more depressed over the past several weeks and was admitted after a suicide attempt. You estimate that you will have her in group for 1 week. You would like to see her mood change in that week. Write an occupation-based goal that will indicate an improved mood.

   C: _____
      (Client will perform)

   O: _____
      (Occupation)

   A: _____
      (Assist level)

   S: _____
      (Specific conditions)

   T: _____
      (Timeline—by when?)

Chapter 7

Writing the "S"—Subjective

The first section of the SOAP note contains **subjective** information obtained from the client, giving his or her perspective on his or her condition or treatment. Subjective data are information that cannot be verified or measured during the treatment session. In this section, the therapist records the client's report of limitations, concerns, and problems, as well as what the client said that was relevant to treatment, such as significant complaints of pain; fatigue; or other expressions of feelings, attitudes, concerns, goals, and plans. When direct quotes are used in the subjective sections of the SOAP note, it is understood that the statement came from the individual receiving therapy unless otherwise stated.

The information obtained from the client will be of greater significance and relevance to the rest of your note if it is specific rather than general in nature. For instance, if the client tells you, "My shoulder hurts," you may question him further, asking him, "Where does it hurt?" or "When does it hurt?" so your note can communicate more detailed information on his condition. You may either use a direct quote or summarize what the client has said, so his description might be written as:

> *Client reports Ⓡ shoulder pain when he tries to put his shirt on.*
> or
> *Client states, "My right shoulder hurts when I try to put my shirt on."*

EXAMPLES OF "S" STATEMENTS

+ *"I don't need therapy."*
+ *Resident reports pain in Ⓡ shoulder when reaching up to comb hair.*
+ *Patient asked for help when it was needed during the session.*
+ *Client reports, "I keep blowing up at home and yelling at everyone, and I don't know what to do about it."*
+ *"I can't wash the dishes or zip my coat."*
+ *Veteran reports that his fingers "feel kind of dead."*
+ *Pt. reported that he needed to go meet someone and get to work when the session began. When asked questions such as "Can you hear me?" he often responded, "I need to go."*
+ *Resident reports he feels "pretty good" now and his goal is to "get back as natural" as he can.*
+ *Consumer reports being fearful of leaving her home.*
+ *Client reports that his doctor has ordered "some home care for a few days to work on transfers."*
+ *Client reported that her shoulders feel better after taping. "My short-term goal is to be able to write, and my long-term goal is to return to work."*

Gateley CA, Borcherding S. *Documentation Manual for Occupational Therapy: Writing SOAP Notes, 3rd Edition* (pp. 63-70)
© 2012 SLACK Incorporated

- *Martha called the emergency room last night to report a burning sensation in her "gut," which made her afraid she was going to die. Today she reports that she has been worrying about dying and has not showered since the day before yesterday.*

- *Resident reports being able to bathe and dress self Ⓘ, but does not open dresser drawers and closet doors due to a recent fall from opening a dresser drawer that resulted in a hip fx. She was able to state the correct day and month when asked.*

- *Pt. commented that she used to use her Ⓛ hand to hold a cup but now is unable to do so. Pt. also complained of soreness in Ⓛ shoulder and inquired about finding a student to assist her at home upon discharge.*

- *Client stated that she has experienced several episodes of bladder incontinence when trying to make it to the bathroom.*

- *Consumer reports that the hardest feelings for her to deal with are worry and fear about her physical problems, which might go undetected. She reports being unable to function at home (cannot cook, keep house, or do laundry) when she is "sick with depression," but wants to do these things again. Consumer reports that exercise, prayer, and volunteer work are her primary coping strategies, and that she would like to learn more about relaxation techniques.*

- *Student reports frustration with handwriting tasks, stating, "I'm just no good at it. I hate writing!"*

As part of the initial evaluation process, an occupational therapist works toward establishing a collaborative relationship with the client by interviewing the client about his or her concerns and priorities and developing an **occupational profile**. The occupational profile is the "summary of information that describes the client's occupational history and experiences, patterns of daily living, interests, values, and needs" (AOTA, 2008b, p. 649). Additional information for the occupational profile may be gathered from discussions with family or caregivers, and through review of existing health records. In an evaluation note, the "S" may contain all or part of the client's occupational profile.

For example:

- *Client reports that she was admitted after a fall that resulted in confusion and left-sided weakness. Prior to admission, she was living alone in a one-story home and was Ⓘ in all ADLs. She reports that she is a retired librarian, widowed 10 years ago. She says she values her independence and fully intends to return to her own home. She reports that her activities are primarily sedentary, including sewing, reading, and playing cards with friends. She says her daughter lives two blocks away and provides transportation when needed.*

Another example:

- *The client talked about his current symptoms and the events leading up to his hospitalization. He reports losing his job with United Construction after not reporting to work for 2 weeks due to depression, having an argument with his wife, and taking an overdose. He says that he has always "worked construction" and does not know how to do anything else. He reports concerns that his former employer will not give him "a decent reference." He says he really has no leisure interests except "going out drinking with the guys after work" and sometimes going hunting in the fall.*

Sometimes the client is not able to speak or does not make any relevant comments. In such cases, include that information in the "S" section.

For example:

- *Client unable to communicate verbally due to expressive aphasia.*
- *Client did not speak without cueing.*
- *Using her augmentative communication device, pt. reported that she wanted to be able to take care of herself.*
- *Resident does not clearly verbalize during treatment, but smiles and nods appropriately when asked questions.*

Sometimes you will include information that the family or caregiver provided about the client if this is pertinent to the session or the client's progress. This is common when treating infants and very young children.

For example:

- *Mother reports difficulty with diapering and dressing the infant, stating, "He just gets all stiff and arches his back."*
- *Foster parents report that child exhibits excessive energy, constantly running around the house and jumping on furniture. They also report that child is aggressive toward foster siblings and the family pet, and he will not remain seated at mealtimes.*

✦ *Parents report child has difficulty remaining in upright seated position for feeding in standard high chair. "She just falls to the right side."*

While the "S" is primarily reserved for the client's view, occasionally it is acceptable to report comments from caregivers and other professionals if the comments are directly related to the client's occupational therapy services. This allows you to demonstrate the collaborative efforts of the treatment team.

For example:

✦ *Pt. tearful throughout session, with very little verbalization. Social worker reports pt.'s family just informed pt. they cannot care for her at home and that she will have to go to a skilled nursing facility.*

✦ *Classroom teacher reports significant improvement in child's ability to remain seated at desk since implementing use of sensory-cushion in chair to provide additional proprioceptive input. Child states, "I love the bumpy feel of it!"*

✦ *Physical therapist reports patient should use sliding board for all transfers as she is unable to maintain weightbearing precautions for pivot transfers. Patient states, "I can use that board getting from the wheelchair to the bed, but I'm afraid I'll fall off if I use it to get to the toilet."*

✦ *Client reports no difficulty with financial management, but spouse reports multiple errors in bill paying and checkbook management in recent months.*

COMMON ERRORS

NOT USING COMMUNICATION TIME WITH THE CLIENT EFFECTIVELY

The most common error that new therapists make in gathering subjective information is in failing to make good use of time when communicating with the client during treatment sessions. Instead of using the time in therapy to talk socially, a good therapist will use the time to listen effectively and to ask questions that will provide pertinent information about the client's attitudes and concerns. This information can be used to ensure effective treatment as well as appropriate documentation. Instead of talking to your client about the weather or Monday Night Football, why not ask him how he thinks he is doing in therapy or what his feelings are related to his upcoming discharge placement? As therapists gain experience, they begin to use the treatment session to gather relevant data regarding such things as occupational history, functional status, prior level of functioning, motivation, priorities, and family support.

Effective communication and interviewing during treatment sessions can seem just like a conversation on the surface. However, as a skilled therapist, you are directing the conversation to topics that are meaningful to client care rather than allowing it to remain superficial. Use this opportunity to expand your occupational profile of the client and to gather data that are vital to providing the very best occupational therapy possible. In having a conversation with your client, guide the discussion to your client's history, problems, needs, strengths, support systems, living situation, and goals for treatment. Without knowing these things from your client's point of view, you will have difficulty planning effective treatment. When a therapist does not listen effectively during treatment, the "S" may read:

✦ *Client talked about grandchildren visiting*

✦ *Patient reports he is reading a good book.*

While these statements are within the scope of the "S," they are not particularly helpful pieces of information to spend the time and space reporting.

NOT WRITING CONCISE, COHERENT STATEMENTS

The second most common error made by new therapists in writing the subjective section of the note is that of simply listing all remarks that the client makes about his or her condition. For example, during one treatment session, the following subjective information was gathered:

✦ *Client said, "I can't feel anything with my hands."*

✦ *Client stated, "I'm as wobbly as all get out today."*

✦ *Client expressed dizziness after bending down to touch the floor while in a seated position.*

✦ *Client acknowledged improvement in his sitting balance in comparison to the previous week.*

Many of these statements have to do with stability, balance, and safety. Although the quotations are a very objective way of reporting data, and all the statements are relevant to the intervention session, it is more effective to summarize the client's remarks in a concise and coherent manner instead of listing each of these statements separately in the "S" section of the note.

For example:

✦ *Client expressed lack of sensation in both hands and dizziness in sitting position with dynamic movement (a "wobbly" sensation). He also acknowledged improvement in sitting balance since last week.*

✦ *Client acknowledged improved sitting balance compared to previous week. However, he experienced dizziness after bending down while sitting, and reported feeling "wobbly." Client also reported inability to feel anything with his hands.*

In Worksheet 7-1, you will have the opportunity to combine a client's statements into a coherent and concise "S" statement.

WORKSHEET 7-1

Writing Concise, Coherent "S" Statements

1. Mrs. P is recovering from a total hip replacement. During a treatment session, she makes the following statements:
   - "I used that dressing stick and sock aid like you showed me to get dressed without bending down this morning."
   - "My hip doesn't hurt when I stand up or sit down, especially with that new toilet seat you got for me."
   - "It's getting easier for me to get dressed now."
   - "My daughter said they delivered all that bathroom equipment to her house yesterday."

Using these statements, write your own concise and organized version for the "S" portion of the SOAP note:

2. Ryan is a 14-year-old recently admitted to an inpatient adolescent psychiatric unit following an unsuccessful suicide attempt by overdose with his mother's sleeping pills. During a group session he makes the following comments:
   - "I have nothing to live for."
   - "I don't have any friends."
   - "My family would be better off without me anyway."
   - "The teachers at my school all hate me."
   - "Maybe next time I should do it right and just use a gun!"

Using these statements, write your own concise and organized version for the "S" portion of the SOAP note:

WORKSHEET 7-2

Choosing a Subjective Statement

An occupational therapist wrote the following observation after treating Mrs. W, a 62-year-old woman who had a stroke 3 weeks ago:

O: *Client participated in 30-minute OT session in rehab gym for UE activities to ↑ AROM in Ⓡ shoulder, activity tolerance, UE strength, and dynamic standing balance, in order to ↑ independence in ADL tasks.*

ADLs: In room, client was instructed in safety techniques and adaptive equipment use in toileting. Client needs Ⓑ grab bars in bathroom for safe sit → stand transition during toileting. Client attempted to stand by pulling on walker and one grab bar. Client was educated on safety issues and the use of Ⓑ grab bars; she verbalized understanding of recommendations.

Performance Skills: Client required CGA for balance during sit ↔ stand. In order to address activity tolerance, dynamic standing balance, and ↑ AROM in Ⓡ shoulder, client moved canned goods from counter to cupboard for 5 minutes before needing a 2-minute seated rest break. After resting, she participated in activities to ↑ dynamic standing balance by pouring liquid from a pitcher while standing with CGA for balance. After a 1-minute seated rest, client continued activities to ↑ dynamic standing balance and safety by retrieving objects from floor using reacher while ambulating c̄ wheeled walker and CGA.

Client Factors: Ⓡ shoulder abduction AROM < 90°. Ⓡ shoulder abduction PROM WFL.

The treatment session included all of the following. Which would be best to use as the subjective portion of the SOAP note?

1. *Client was very cooperative and engaged in social conversation throughout the tx. session.*
2. *Client remarked that her grandson will be coming to visit later in the week, and that she will be very glad to see him.*
3. *Client reports that she feels "pretty good" today.*
4. *Client says she has difficulty moving Ⓡ UE, although she does not know why it will not move. She reports, "It really doesn't hurt. It's just tight."*
5. *Nursing staff report client is incontinent at night.*

Writing the "O"—Objective

The next part of the note is the **objective** section, where you will record all measurable, quantifiable, and observable data obtained during the treatment session. In this section, you will present a picture of the intervention session you have provided. Once you start looking at things with your professional eyes, they can look quite different. Instead of seeing a child playing with a toy, now you begin to note the child's asymmetrical posture, his bilateral hand use, his difficulty crossing midline, and his grasp and pinch patterns. The trick in writing the "O" is knowing what kind of material to include and what to omit. At first your "O" may tend to be longer than that of an experienced therapist, but with time you will learn to write notes that are both complete and concise.

THREE STEPS TO WRITING GOOD OBSERVATIONS

There are three important steps to remember when writing the "O" section of your SOAP note:
1. Begin with a statement about the setting and purpose of the treatment session.
2. Follow the opening statement with a summary of what you observed.
3. Be professional, concise, and specific.
We will look at each of these steps more in depth in the following sections.

STEP 1: BEGIN WITH A STATEMENT ABOUT THE SETTING AND PURPOSE OF THE TREATMENT SESSION

This opening statement gives the reader an introduction to the remainder of the "O" section. It explains the "where," "what," "how long," and "why" about the client's occupational therapy services. Your documentation is the basis for answering any questions about the services that a client received. In Chapter 3, you learned about CPT codes. Most CPT codes are based on the number of minutes of each specific service the client received. Facilities that do not charge for occupational therapy by the number of minutes provided may not require that you document the length of the treatment session.

Sames (2010) suggested that practitioners move away from passive terminology that the client was "seen" in occupational therapy, and instead state that the client "participated in" the occupational therapy session (p. 10). This distinction is important since funding sources want evidence that the client is actively participating in the habilitation or rehabilitation process.

> If you are utilizing "occupation-based interventions" (AOTA, 2008b, p. 653), use the following format for your opening statement:
>
> Client participated in ___ -minute OT session _____ for _____.
>   #   in what setting   occupation-based intervention

Gateley CA, Borcherding S. *Documentation Manual for Occupational Therapy: Writing SOAP Notes, 3rd Edition* (pp. 71-88)
© 2012 SLACK Incorporated

For example:

✦ *Client participated in 45-minute OT session in rehab kitchen for meal-preparation activity.*

✦ *Consumer participated in 2-hour supervised outing involving use of public transportation system for community mobility.*

✦ *Patient participated in 30-minute OT session in hospital room for completion of morning bathing, dressing, and grooming routine using adaptive equipment.*

If the session focuses on "purposeful activity" or "preparatory methods" (AOTA, 2008b, p. 653), then add a reference to the relevant area of occupation in the opening statement:

Client participated in ___ -minute OT session _____ for _____ for _____ .
       #   in what setting   intervention   what expected occupational gain

---

For example:

✦ *Child participated in 30-minute OT session in outpatient clinic focusing on improving postural control and Ⓑ UE coordination for increased success in play activities.*

✦ *Student participated in 30-minute OT session in classroom with focus on improving sensory processing and selective attention needed for engagement in classroom activities.*

✦ *Client participated in 30-minute OT session in room for skilled instruction in energy conservation during IADL activities.*

✦ *Joe participated in role-play activity during 30-minute assertion group in order to explore alternative ways to meet his social needs.*

✦ *Patient participated in 30-minute OT session in rehab gym bathroom to practice transfer using tub bench for increased safety and independence during bathing.*

✦ *Client participated in 30-minute OT session in outpatient hand clinic to address Ⓡ hand strengthening and scar desensitization in preparation for return to construction work.*

✦ *Resident participated in 20-minute OT session at sink for instruction on adaptive strategies for grooming Ⓘ.*

✦ *Child participated in 30-minute OT session in therapy room to ↑ strength and tone needed to improve handwriting at school.*

It is essential that you show **the need for your skill as an OT** in this opening statement. So rather than saying, *"Client participated in 45-minute OT session at bedside for ADL training,"* instead you might say:

✦ *Client participated in 45-minute OT session at bedside for skilled instruction in compensatory dressing techniques.*

✦ *Resident participated in 45-minute OT session at bedside for skilled instruction in use of adaptive equipment to increase safety during ADL tasks.*

✦ *Veteran participated in 45-minute OT session at bedside to facilitate attention to Ⓛ side during self-care activities.*

STEP 2: FOLLOW THE OPENING STATEMENT WITH A SUMMARY OF WHAT YOU OBSERVED

After you have established the setting and purpose, you will discuss the interventions that were completed and the client's response to those interventions. There are different ways that are acceptable in organizing the information of the "O":

✦ *Chronologically*: Discuss each treatment event in the order it occurred during the treatment session.

✦ *Categorically*: Organize the information according to categories. The categories you select will vary depending on the client and the purpose of the treatment session. You can refer to the *Framework-II* (AOTA, 2008b) for potential categories. For example, it may be helpful to organize the objective information by areas of occupation, client factors, or performance skills.

• Areas of occupation (e.g., ADLs, IADLs, work, social interaction)

⬥ Note how each of the performance skills and client factors observed impact performance in the relevant areas of occupation. Include assist levels and set-up required, adaptive equipment or techniques used, types of cueing provided, caregiver education, related positioning and mobility issues, and client's response to the treatment provided. Describe consumer's awareness of others in group, initiation of conversation, and interaction with peers in a group setting.

- Client factors (e.g., ROM, strength, edema, sensation)
  ◦ Provide specific measurements such as girth or volumetric measurements for edema, grip and pinch strength, PROM and AROM, and type of sensation that is intact or impaired.
- Performance skills (e.g., balance, coordination, cognition, behavior)
  ◦ Note whether balance was static or dynamic. Consider whether the client leans in one direction, has rotated posture, or uneven weight distribution. Describe hand dominance, types of prehension used, purposeful grasp and release, and gross motor versus fine motor ability. Report on orientation, task initiation, ability to stay on task, sequencing, judgment, and ability to follow directions. Document client's agitation, lethargy, affect, compulsivity, anxiety, or demanding behaviors.

Let's take a look at a few examples of the different ways to organize the "O."

Chronologically

One way to organize the "O" section of your SOAP note is to document events in the order in which they happened during the treatment session. Think of this method as giving the reader a "play-by-play" of the session.

For example:

✦ *Client participated in anger management group for 45 minutes today to improve social interaction skills and ability to maintain employment. Client initially required verbal prompting from nursing staff and security aides to attend group. He displayed displeasure at being asked to attend the group by using profanity. During the group, client related 2 instances in which individuals on the unit consistently bother him, and discussed the way he usually handles the situation. Peer feedback was given on other possible ways he might handle the situation. Client indicated that he would consider these alternatives next time a bothersome situation arises.*

✦ *Client participated in 30-minute evaluation in OT clinic for assessment of low back pain and instruction in proper body mechanics during IADLs. Client was observed to sit with her weight shifted to her ⓛ hip. Client demonstrated the way she usually removes items from the refrigerator, washes dishes, cleans the floors, and lifts. She was then instructed in proper body mechanics for completing IADL tasks including using a golfer's lift, squats, stepping toward the item she wished to retrieve, facing the load, and keeping it close to her body. Client demonstrated these techniques with minimal verbal cues and was provided with educational handouts to remind her of correct positioning.*

Categorically

Alternately, you may choose to organize your information into categories. When categorizing your information, choose categories that make sense for your note. For example, suppose that today you saw a client in the kitchen for a cooking session in preparation for discharge. She plans to cook when she returns home, but you are not certain of her safety or her ability to perform all the steps of the activity from her chair. You wonder if her strength, activity tolerance, and ability to use her involved hand and arm are sufficient for cooking, and you also want to assess her judgment and ability to problem solve. You therefore choose the following categories, using a combination of client factors and performance skills:

✦ Functional mobility
✦ UE range and strength
✦ Hand function and strength
✦ Activity tolerance
✦ Cognition

Your note might look like this:

O: *Client participated in 1-hr OT session in clinic kitchen for skilled instruction in compensatory techniques for safe and independent cooking.*
  ***Functional Mobility**: Client maneuvered throughout kitchen in w/c with verbal cues to place w/c in appropriate position for reaching objects in kitchen. Client required min Ⓐ in stabilizing items while transporting them in lap and maneuvering w/c simultaneously.*
  ***UE ROM and Strength**: WFL for reaching items in drawers, opening oven door, and putting dishes in the sink Ⓘ. UE strength adequate for opening refrigerator door and stirring batter Ⓘ. Client required min Ⓐ in opening a plastic storage container.*

Hand Function and Strength: *Adequate for unscrewing lids, cracking egg, and opening muffin box* Ⓘ. *Client able to use necessary tools for carrying out task* Ⓘ. *Client able to set oven dial and put muffins in oven* Ⓘ.

Activity Tolerance: *Client* Ⓘ *took a 3-minute break after ~ 20 minutes of activity.*

Cognition: *Client able to respond to verbal instruction and questions with correct response 3/3 times. Client said that she did not think it would be safe for her to take the muffins out of the oven. Client able to problem solve* Ⓘ *about repositioning her w/c 75% of tx. time.*

Let's look at another example of a note organized by category. Suppose you work in a school setting and you have a child on your caseload who has been receiving occupational therapy services on a consultative basis one time monthly. During your monthly visit, you consult with the classroom teacher and the child's paraprofessional and observe the child in the classroom. While the child's handwriting performance and ability to meet classroom expectations without disruptive behaviors appear much improved following previous OT recommendations, staff report a new concern that the child is displaying aggression toward classmates when going through the lunch line. You then observe the child during lunch and make recommendations to the teacher and paraprofessional. Your note might look like this:

O: *30-minute monthly consultation completed this date including observation of student in classroom and cafeteria, and recommendations to teacher and paraprofessional to help improve child's ability to participate effectively during lunch.*

Classroom Observations: *Lucas demonstrated ability to remain seated at desk to complete worksheet for 8 minutes while wearing weighted vest for increased proprioception. He is now able to write all letters of the alphabet legibly using adaptive paper with alternating highlighted lines and a rubber pencil grip.*

Cafeteria Observations: *Lucas exhibited verbal and physical aggression (pushing) toward classmate on two separate occasions when inadvertently bumped in line. Follow-up questioning with Lucas indicates that he perceives unexpected touch as "painful."*

Staff Education: *Classroom teacher and Lucas' paraprofessional were educated regarding sensory processing deficits related to unexpected touch. Recommendation was made to either allow Lucas to leave classroom a few minutes early to go to cafeteria or to have him stand at the beginning or end of the line to reduce the chances of classmates bumping into him. Staff verbalized understanding and plan to implement suggestions tomorrow.*

You must realize that there is no "right" list of categories to use. Use what makes sense for the individual client and situation. Worksheet 8-1 will give you the opportunity to rewrite a chronologically organized note into categories.

STEP 3: BE PROFESSIONAL, CONCISE, AND SPECIFIC

The "O" section does not need to be written in complete sentences. Give complete information in the most concise form possible. Some details **must** be included. For example, ROM must be specified as active, passive, or assistive and must indicate the joint at which the movement occurred. You must indicate Ⓡ, Ⓛ, or Ⓑ when discussing UEs or LEs. You must specify the level of assistance that was provided. Below are some examples of wording change that make your documentation more professional, concise, and specific.

Rather than saying: *Resident flopped down onto the bed short of breath, closed her eyes, and moaned. Resident laid in bed with min* Ⓐ *to position herself.*

You might say: *Resident observed to be fatigued and SOB following tx. session and required min* Ⓐ *for positioning in bed.*

Rather than saying: *Veteran had to use a trapeze to sit up.*

You might say: *Supine → sit using trapeze.*

Rather than saying: *Client put the board in place to make a sliding board transfer.*

You might say: *Client positioned sliding board for transfer.*

When you are documenting test results, it is helpful to put them into a chart like the following one, rather than burying them in narrative:

Ⓛ Hand Sensation	
Hot/Cold	Intact
Sharp/Dull	Impaired over volar surface; intact over dorsal surface
Stereognosis	Absent

When you are first learning to write client observations, it is hard to decide what to include and what to leave out. At first, it is better to include too much data rather than taking a chance of omitting something important. As your observational skills become more refined, it will become second nature to include all the important data, and the "O" section of your notes will begin to be more concise. Here is a client observation written by an inexperienced therapist. In an effort to include all the necessary data, she wrote a note that was too wordy.

O: *Client participated in 30 minutes of Ⓡ UE strengthening in therapy gym in order to prevent future shoulder dislocation. Client was asked to clasp hands together and raise arms above head x 30. Client was then instructed to cross her midline and touch her opposite shoulder with Ⓡ UE. Client required 6 rest periods for completion. Client completed tasks Ⓘ. Client was then introduced to weight and pulley system. Client was asked to specify how much weight she thought she could do. She responded with 5#. Client did 30 repetitions of the pulley system with 5# in shoulder flexion to strengthen her rotator cuff to decrease the probability of dislocating her shoulder again. After strengthening exercise, client had 3 heat packs applied to shoulder to decrease pain.*

A more experienced therapist might have written:

O: *Client participated in 30 minutes of Ⓡ UE strengthening in therapy gym in order to prevent future shoulder dislocation. Client completed the following:*

  ❖ *Ⓑ clasped-hand shoulder flexion and extension x 30 repetitions*
  ❖ *Horizontal adduction Ⓡ hand to Ⓛ shoulder x 30 repetitions*
  ❖ *Ⓡ shoulder flexion pulleys with 5# wt. x 30 repetitions*

  3 hot packs applied to Ⓡ shoulder to ↓ pain after tx.

You will notice, however, that there is another problem with this note besides the fact that the original note is wordy. It also sounds like a physical therapy note rather than an occupational therapy note. This note needs to have a functional component added in the opening statement of the "O" section. A statement from the client in the "S" about what she is unable to do with an injured rotator cuff and a statement in the "A" and/or "P" indicating functional problems/goals would suffice to make it a good occupational therapy note.

Notice that being more concise means knowing what information can be omitted without compromising the quality of the observation. It is possible to be too concise, omitting necessary information. For example, consider the following "O" from a community mental health center evaluation:

O: *Client evaluated in office using COPM. Client required 45 minutes to complete COPM. Client responded to directive questions regarding self-care, productivity, and leisure.*

This "O" does not provide much information. When additional information is added, we learn much more about the evaluation session with this client:

O: *Client participated in evaluation in office using the Canadian Occupational Performance Measure (COPM), which she completed in 45 minutes. She arrived 45 minutes late to the appointment, well groomed and neatly dressed. Questions regarding productivity and leisure were answered with clear enunciation and animated tone, but questions about self-care (particularly those about scar management) were declined or given short answers with sad tone and no eye contact. Client frequently touched scars on trunk during the evaluation.*

It is a matter of balancing the need to be complete with the need to be concise when writing the "O." Worksheet 8-2 will give you an opportunity to make an observation more concise without losing any of its informational content.

TIPS FOR MAKING YOUR DOCUMENTATION SOUND MORE PROFESSIONAL

There are several ways to make your documentation sound professional. Here are some tips to remember when writing your note:

✦ Focus on occupation.
✦ Focus on the client's response to the treatment provided rather than on what the therapist did.

+ Write from the client's point of view, leaving yourself out.
+ Be specific about assist levels.
+ Avoid making a list of actions and assist levels.
+ De-emphasize the treatment media.
+ Make it clear that you were not just a passive observer in the session.
+ Avoid judging the client.
+ Use only standard abbreviations.

Let's look at some examples of each of these recommendations.

FOCUS ON OCCUPATION

Make certain that occupation is integral to the note. In a treatment session devoted to self-care activities, function is obvious. However, in a session devoted to addressing client factors such as strength or endurance, in a session where modalities are used, or in a cotreatment session, function must be addressed separately in order to justify skilled occupational therapy. For example, although the note below is an observation of a session that was devoted to performance components, it contains a statement about the functional intent of the exercises.

O: *Veteran participated in 30-minute OT session in room for AROM and strengthening of Ⓛ UE in order to regain ability to dress self. Client performed self-ranging exercises from standing and seated position with SBA for balance and verbal instructions to correct errors. Client required 5 verbal cues to reach higher with Ⓛ UE during shoulder flexion AROM.*

FOCUS ON THE CLIENT'S RESPONSE TO THE TREATMENT PROVIDED

Rather than saying: *Client was reminded about hip precautions.*

You might say: *Client required 4 verbal cues to keep hip in correct alignment when donning shoes.*

Rather than saying: *Client was asked orientation questions pertaining to the time of day.*

You might say: *When verbally cued to look at watch, client was unable to correctly identify time.*

Rather than saying: *Client reminded to relax.*

You might say: *UE tone moderately increased but relaxes with verbal cue.*

Rather than saying: *Child was given a puzzle to play with.*

You might say: *Child able to place simple shapes into inset puzzle with min Ⓐ to reposition pieces.*

WRITE FROM THE CLIENT'S POINT OF VIEW

The focus of good professional writing is always on the client. Turn your sentences around so that the client is the subject of your sentence.

Rather than saying: *The OT put the client's shoes on for him.*

You might say: *Client unable to don shoes.*

Rather than saying: *OT instructed the client and family in energy conservation techniques.*

You might say: *Client and family instructed in energy conservation techniques and demonstrated understanding by incorporating techniques during ADL tasks.*

BE SPECIFIC ABOUT ASSIST LEVELS

When documenting assist levels, be sure to note what part of the activity the client needed physical assistance or verbal cues to perform.

For example:
+ *Veteran doffed night garment with min Ⓐ **to untie strings in back**.*

+ *Child needed HOH assist **for accuracy** when cutting with scissors.*
+ *Client required verbal cues **to sit down** for safety when doffing hosiery.*
+ *Consumer able to follow bus schedule with min verbal cues **to identify correct time**.*
+ *Resident completed supine → sit in bed with min verbal cues **to roll to Ⓡ side**.*
+ *When transitioning stand → w/c using a standard walker, pt. required min physical Ⓐ and min verbal cues **to bring walker completely back to w/c**.*
+ *Infant able to roll supine to prone with min tactile cues **to initiate movement**.*
+ *Pt. completed standing pivot transfer with verbal cues **on hand placement needed for safety**.*
+ *Client required mod Ⓐ **to follow total hip precautions** while washing lower legs and feet with long-handled sponge.*

Worksheet 8-3 will give you practice in being specific about assist levels.

AVOID MAKING A LIST OF ACTIONS AND ASSIST LEVELS

In trying to be concise, sometimes inexperienced therapists make the mistake of writing an "O" that contains only a list of actions with assist levels. While this is a common error, it is **incorrect**. Simply writing a list of activities or assist levels **does not show the skilled OT** being provided. Consider this OT's observation:

O: *Client participated in 1-hr OT session in shower room to ↑ activity tolerance and improve balance during showering. Client was shown a smaller shower that simulated her home shower, in order to prepare for discharge in 1 week.*
Client Ox4.
Client required min Ⓐ with verbal cues to sit in w/c to doff hosiery and to dry off Ⓑ LEs.
Client spontaneously rinsed soap off hands before gripping grab bar while showering.
Client used walker going to and coming from shower room.
Client tolerated standing Ⓘ during entire shower.
Client instructed in home showering.

Now let's take a look at the same observation, rewritten in a more useful format:

O: *Client participated in 1-hr OT session in shower room to ↑ activity tolerance and improve balance during showering. Client completed shower in smaller shower stall that simulates her home shower in order to prepare her for safe and Ⓘ showering after discharge in 1 week.*
***Functional Mobility**: Pt ambulated to/from shower room and completed standing portion of dressing/undressing with modified Ⓘ using standard walker for stability.*
***Cognition**: Client oriented x 4.*
***ADLs**: Client required min Ⓐ and verbal cues to sit down in order to doff hosiery and to dry Ⓑ LEs safely. Client rinsed soap off hands s̄ verbal cues prior to gripping grab bar during shower. Client tolerated standing Ⓘ ~ 5 minutes during shower s̄ SOB. Client received skilled instruction in safe technique to use in her single shower stall and recommendations were provided re: grab bar placement.*

DE-EMPHASIZE THE TREATMENT MEDIA

In order to improve a client's performance skills, you may use various media, such as equipment or activities that will help the client reach functional goals. However, when documenting your observations of these treatment sessions, you should de-emphasize the media used and focus instead on the performance skills. For example, an inexperienced therapist might write the following:

Client worked on placing pegs into a pegboard.

This statement may accurately describe what a casual observer would see, but as a trained professional, you need to look beyond the media used and see what the client was really accomplishing. The media used here are pegs and a pegboard, but what is the performance skill? Placing pegs into a pegboard is not a skill this client needs in order to be able to care for herself. However, the performance skills she practices during this activity may well be crucial to achieving independence. Suppose the therapist had written:

Client worked on tripod pinch using pegs and a pegboard.

Notice that in this example the therapist did not simply add the performance skill to the statement "*Client worked on placing pegs into pegboard to increase tripod pinch*," but actually turned the sentence around so that the tripod pinch received the emphasis and the media was mentioned only for clarification. Suppose the therapist had written:

> *Client worked on tripod pinch in order to be able to grasp objects needed for ADL tasks.*

In this case mention of the media becomes optional. She could also have written:

> *Client worked on tripod pinch using pegs and a pegboard in order to be able to grasp objects needed for ADL tasks.*

Which of the three preceding examples do you think best describes the skilled instruction that is occurring in this treatment session? This may seem like a minor distinction, but it is important in demonstrating the need for skilled OT and the emphasis on functional outcomes in therapy.

One of the most common errors among inexperienced OTs is focusing on the media used rather than on the performance skill and area of occupation that are being improved by use of the media. Consider this OT's observation:

O: *Client participated in 30-minute OT session at outpatient rehab clinic for standing balance activities. Client used (R) UE to hit balloon and was able to reach to (R) and (L) sides approximately 7 out of 10 tries. Activity was continued for 3 minutes. Client requested rest break and sat for 30 seconds. Client then stood with mod (A) to walker and hit balloon with (L) UE for 3 minutes. Client was able to hit balloon approximately 6 out of 10 times and spontaneously switched to (R) hand x 2 when balloon was to her far right. Client sat for another break and to switch activities. Client stood with CGA to toss beanbags with (R) hand for 4 minutes. Client scored 240 points with (R) hand by throwing beanbags at target. Once all beanbags were thrown, client sat for a 30-second break. Client stood with CGA for balance to toss beanbags with (L) hand for 30 seconds. Client scored 150 points with (L) hand by throwing beanbags at scoring target. Once all beanbags were thrown, client sat and session was ended.*

When this note is rewritten to focus on the performance skills, notice the difference in professionalism and the way the note reads:

O: *Client participated in 30-minute OT session at outpatient rehab clinic to address standing balance needed for ADL and IADL tasks. Pt stood to walker with mod (A) for dynamic standing balance necessary for (I) showering, using a balloon toss activity. Client held walker with (L) hand and used (R) UE to reach both (R) and (L) sides approximately 7/10 attempts. Client sustained activity for 3 minutes continuously before requiring a 30-second seated rest break. Client stood to walker again with mod (A) for 3 minutes of continuous activity involving weight shifting and balance. Client demonstrated ability to reach to (R) and (L) sides to reach for moving object approximately 6/10 times. Client demonstrated ability to spontaneously weight shift 2 times to reach object. Client required another 30-second seated rest before next activity. Client worked on dynamic standing balance using beanbag toss activity with target. Client stood to walker for 4 minutes of dynamic balance activity with CGA, then sat for a 30-second rest. Client stood again with CGA for 3 ½ minutes of continuous dynamic balance activity.*

Refer to Worksheet 8-4 for practice in de-emphasizing the treatment media.

MAKE IT CLEAR THAT YOU WERE NOT JUST A PASSIVE OBSERVER IN THE SESSION

This will be a critical factor in reimbursement. We do not get paid to **watch** a client do something. To show that the skill of an occupational therapist is needed, you must be actively involved in intervention, such as evaluating or modifying the activity; otherwise it will be considered unskilled.

Rather than saying: *Client compensated for shoulder flexion by leaning forward with entire body during prehension activities.*

You might say: *Client required skilled instruction to avoid compensation at the shoulder during prehension activities.*

Rather than saying: *Client performed Home Exercise Program.*

You might say: *Home Exercise Program was observed for accurate movement patterns and updated to accommodate for progress.*

AVOID JUDGING THE CLIENT

Rather than saying: *Client was compliant.* or *Client was cooperative.*

You might say: *Client demonstrated ability to follow 3-step directions and sequence WFL.*

When you are working with a client who is difficult or whose opinions and behavior you do not agree with, it is easy to judge the client and to reflect your judgments in your observation. Below is a note written by a student who was in a difficult situation. The client "went off on" the student, refusing a sponge bath, lying about having already bathed, throwing her washcloth across the room so the student would have to pick it up, refusing to put on her slacks, and announcing that therapy was "stupid." In spite of all this, the student wrote an observation that was nonjudgmental of the client:

> *Client required max encouragement to participate in 30-minute therapy session this AM. Client completed sit → stand & ambulated to sink Ⓘ. Client Ⓘ at sink c̄ simulated bathing activity using long-handled sponge. Client Ⓘ retrieved washcloth from floor using a reacher. Client able to don/doff socks and shoes c̄ adaptive equipment p̄ set-up. Client retrieved gown and socks Ⓘ c̄ reacher. Client declined to don slacks.*

USE ONLY STANDARD ABBREVIATIONS

You may use the abbreviations **approved by your facility**. Please note that the list of abbreviations provided in Chapter 4 is for purposes of learning to document using the exercises in this workbook. Do not use any other abbreviations even if they seem common to you. If you try to read a note containing abbreviations with which you are unfamiliar, you will understand instantly how important this is. Remember that your documentation must be read by those unfamiliar with the "shorthand" that health professionals use so freely. Suppose your chart is being read by someone who is from a different background, such as an insurance clerk, attorney, or committee at the Lion's Club who is considering funding a piece of equipment for your client. To make your note understandable to all readers, be judicious in applying abbreviations and keep them very standard. A good rule to follow: **When in doubt, write it out!**

SUMMARY

Good documentation is based on accurate observation, which is based on knowing what to look for. For an experienced therapist, this becomes second nature. For a student therapist, it is helpful to review the lists in this manual and to check your observations against what your supervising therapist observed during the treatment session to be sure you are noticing the items that matter most.

WORKSHEET 8-1

Using Categories

Consider the following chronological observation:

O: *Child participated in 60-minute OT session at daycare to address feeding skills and reach/grasp/release during play. With min Ⓐ for facilitation of movement at elbow, child demonstrated ability to use Ⓛ UE to reach, grasp, and release 5 objects with 1-2 verbal cues per object and restriction of Ⓡ UE movement. Child was able to feed self Ⓘ $\bar{c}$ ~50% spillage, but demonstrated significant limitations in chewing action $\bar{p}$ ~3 rotary chews & swallowing ~90% of food $\bar{s}$ chewing. Child required verbal cues throughout session to maintain attention to task. Child wore soft spica thumb splint for entire session.*

How would you divide this information into categories to make it easier to read? Choose 3 to 4 categories and redistribute the information above into the categories you have chosen.

WORKSHEET 8-2

Being More Concise

Revise the following note to be complete but more concise.

O: *Pt. participated in 60-minute OT session bedside to complete morning ADL routine. Pt. ambulated ~36 inches to shower c̄ SBA for safety. Pt. instructed to complete shower while sitting. Pt performed shower c̄ SBA to manage IV line. Pt. able to wash upper and lower body ① and dry entire body after completing shower. Pt. required ~20 minutes to complete shower. Pt. then ambulated ~36 inches to chair and sat. Pt. needed verbal cues to remain seated while donning underwear and pants. Pt. able to dress upper body ① and lower body p̄ verbal cues for sitting. Pt. demonstrated good sitting balance, but needed SBA for standing balance. Following shower, client stated he would like to take a nap and was assisted back to bed.*

WORKSHEET 8-3

Being Specific About Assist Levels

When noting assist levels in your observation, it is not enough to note just the level of assistance required. You also need to note the part of the task that required assistance.

For example:

✦ *Resident donned pants with min Ⓐ **to pull up over hips**.*

✦ *Client propelled w/c from room to OT clinic but required verbal cues **to avoid running into other clients**.*

Rewrite the statements below to provide a part of the task that required assistance. Since you have not seen the client, you cannot know what part really required assistance. In the real world of professional behavior, making things up is fraud, so please keep in mind that the client you are about to imagine is just an exercise in creativity. For this exercise, you will create a client in your mind and imagine that client doing the task described. As you watch your client in your mind, notice what parts of the task required assistance, and modify the sentences below accordingly.

1. *Client completed supine → sit with min Ⓐ; bed → w/c with mod Ⓐ.*

2. *Client required SBA in transferring w/c ↔ toilet.*

3. *Client retrieved garments from low drawers with min Ⓐ.*

4. *Client required max Ⓐ to brush hair.*

5. *Client completed dressing, toileting, and hygiene with min Ⓐ.*

WORKSHEET 8-4

De-emphasizing the Treatment Media

Rewrite the following statements to emphasize the skilled OT that is actually occurring in the treatment session.

1. *Client played catch using Ⓑ UEs to facilitate grasp and release patterns.*

2. *Resident put dirt into pot to halfway point, added seedling, and filled remainder of pot with dirt transferred by cup. Resident completed 3 more pots while standing 8 minutes before requiring a 5-minute rest. Resident resumed standing position to water completed pots for approximately 5 minutes.*

3. *Client painted some suncatchers in crafts group to be able to see that she could do something successfully.*

Writing the "A"—Assessment

The third section of the note is the **assessment**, which contains the therapist's appraisal of the client's progress, occupational limitations, and expected benefit from OT intervention. In the assessment section of the note, you will use your clinical reasoning to interpret the meaning of the data you have presented in the "S" and "O" sections. You will describe what it means in your professional judgment and its potential impact on the client's ability to engage in meaningful occupation.

In the assessment section of your note, you will primarily note the 3 Ps: **problems**, **progress**, and rehab **potential**. You might also point out inconsistencies, discuss emotional components, or present some reason that something was not done as planned. Finally, the assessment section is where you justify continuation of OT services.

> The assessment is the "heart" of your note. If you could write only six lines, the assessment section of your note would contain the six lines you would choose. This is the section that demonstrates your clinical reasoning as an occupational therapy practitioner.

ASSESSING THE DATA

To assess the data, go sentence by sentence through the information presented in the "S" and the "O," asking yourself what it means for the client's ability to engage in meaningful occupation. Note what problems, progress, and potential for rehabilitation you see.

PROBLEMS

Some notes will show progress and/or rehab potential and some will not, but almost all notes will show problem areas. The problem areas are what keep a client in active treatment. Problems may include the following:

✦ Safety risks:
  • *Attempt to stand without locking w/c brakes raises safety concerns.*
  • *Poor problem solving when using the stove raises safety concerns for staying home alone.*
  • *Limited coping strategies for dealing with stress raise concerns for continuing to demonstrate self-destructive behaviors.*

✦ Inconsistencies between client report and objective findings:
  • *Although client reports anticipating no difficulty in returning to prehospitalization level of homemaking activity, her left-side neglect could cause significant in-home safety risks.*
  • *Although client expresses willingness to do ADL tasks, motor planning problems create a barrier to ADL task performance.*
  • *Although client verbalizes a desire to progress to the next level of responsibility, ↓ behavioral control when reward incentives are unavailable limits this progress.*

Gateley CA, Borcherding S. *Documentation Manual for Occupational Therapy: Writing SOAP Notes, 3rd Edition* (pp. 89-104)
© 2012 SLACK Incorporated

✦ Contributing factors that can be influenced by OT intervention:
- *Left-side weakness interferes with standing balance in tub.*
- *Left-side neglect necessitates verbal cues to attend to left side during ADL tasks.*
- *Deficits in cognitive processing create a need for constant verbal cues to perform kitchen tasks safely.*

The most common problem area that you will be assessing is the impact of a contributing factor on the ability to engage in occupation. When therapists are first learning to write SOAP notes, they may find it difficult to distinguish observations from assessments. There is a formula you can use to write about a problem area that is not within functional limits (WFL), insuring that you are writing an assessment rather than an observation. This formula calls for **making the limiting factor the subject of the sentence**, and then telling how that factor impacts a client's ability to engage in occupation.

Contributing Factor	Impact	Ability to Engage in Occupation

You may want to refer back to Chapter 1 and review the aspects of OT's domain as described in the *Framework-II* (AOTA, 2008b) to identify the contributing factors.

For example:

✦ Client factors: ROM, strength, edema, sensation, etc.
- ***Deficits in UE strength and activity tolerance*** *limit client's ability to complete basic self-care tasks.*
- ***Lack of forearm supination and active elbow flexion against gravity*** *interfere with child's ability to perform age-appropriate developmental play activities.*
- ***Pain in Ⓛ shoulder*** *limits client's ability to carry out child-care and household management tasks.*

✦ Performance skills: Balance, coordination, cognition, behavior, social interaction, etc.
- ***Deficits in attention span*** *make IADLs difficult and potentially unsafe.*
- ***Inability to manage anger*** *results in difficulty finding work and establishing successful intimate relationships.*
- ***Decreased fine motor coordination*** *impacts child's ability to write name.*

✦ Performance patterns: Habits, routines, etc.
- ***Perseveration with lining up toys*** *limits child's social interaction with peers at school.*
- *Client's* ***gambling habits*** *result in lack of financial resources to pay monthly rent.*
- *Client's* ***routine of watching television for 12+ hours daily*** *limits performance of household management tasks.*

✦ Context and environment: Natural environment, built environment, socioeconomic status, social environment, etc.
- ***Extraneous noises in classroom*** *limit child's ability to attend to written work.*
- ***Narrow doorways in home*** *inhibit client's ability to access the bathroom from w/c level for toileting and bathing.*
- ***Lack of financial resources*** *impacts client's ability to purchase clothing necessary to obtain employment.*

✦ Activity demands: Space demands, social demands, sequencing and timing requirements, required body functions and structures, etc.
- ***Need for assistance during multi-step sequences*** *limits independence with self-catheterization.*
- ***One-handedness following traumatic amputation of*** Ⓡ ***hand*** *limits ability to tie shoes.*
- ***Inability to tolerate close proximity of classmates during circle time*** *interferes with child's ability to participate in group classroom activities.*

Notice that in each example given above, the contributing factor is the subject of the sentence, and then it is followed by the negative impact it has on a specific area of occupation. This is not the only way to write an assessment of problem areas, but the formula is a good one when you are first learning. Refer to Worksheet 9-1 for practice using this formula of writing assessment statements.

Note: The assessment section is NOT the place to introduce new data. Do not put anything in your "A" that has not been discussed in the "S" or "O." If you find yourself wanting to make a statement in the "A" that is not supported by the data in your "S" or "O," ask yourself what you might have observed to support the assessment statement. Then decide whether you need to add it to your "S" or "O."

Progress

Think about indications that the OT treatment being provided is effective. What improvements have you observed? This may be progress that you observe within a single session or progress as compared to a previous session. For example:

+ *Weighted utensils decrease intention tremors by ~50% when eating.*
+ *Brady is making progress toward community re-entry as shown by his ability to prepare for an outing, respect rules by following directions, interact socially with staff, and control his behavior ~50% of the time.*
+ *Ten degree ↑ in AROM in (L) elbow this week allows client to don shirt (I).*
+ *Infant's ability to maintain seated position during play indicates improved postural control.*
+ *Patient's ability to attend to ADL tasks for 3 minutes today is significantly improved from baseline attention span of 60 seconds.*
+ *Client's spontaneous participation in group discussion shows good progress in developing social interaction skills.*
+ *Child's improved prehension skills now enable child to zip coat.*

Sometimes progress is indicated by stating that previous goals have been met or modified:

+ *STG #2 (buttoning ½-inch buttons X 3 on shirt) met this week.*
+ *STG #3 upgraded to "complete grooming tasks, <u>standing</u> for at least 3 minutes at sink."*
+ *STG #4 changed to "attend at least 2 group sessions daily."*

Sometimes you may need to explain why there has been a lack of progress:

+ *Patient has become more dependent in ADL tasks this week due to acute infection.*
+ *Client's attendance of therapy sessions this month has been sporadic due to spouse being terminally ill.*
+ *Child's progress toward handwriting goals has been limited due to recent (R) radius fracture and casting of dominant (R) UE.*
+ *Patient's ability to remain alert during session was impaired due to anesthesia from medical procedure earlier this date.*

Potential

In addition to problems and progress, the "A" section is also where you should comment on the client's potential for success in rehabilitation:

+ *Ability to understand instructions and desire to return to living independently indicate good potential to return to prior living situation.*
+ *Patient's ability to recall and demonstrate 3/3 hip precautions shows good potential to follow hip precautions after discharge.*
+ *Patient's intact cognitive skills indicate good potential for learning compensatory strategies for ADLs and IADLs.*
+ *Participation in groups, including not interrupting, asking questions appropriately, and sharing experiences, indicates good potential to benefit from psychiatric rehab program.*
+ *Student's progress in ability to use scissors indicates good potential to meet goals stated in IEP.*

Justifying Continuation of Occupational Therapy Services

After you have documented the client's problems, progress, and potential, you should end the "A" section of your note with a justification of continued OT services. One very useful way of justifying continued OT treatment for your client is to end the "A" with the statement *"Client would benefit from..."* and complete the sentence with a justification of continued treatment that requires the skill of an OT practitioner. Not every therapist ends the "A" with this method, but for purposes of learning, we will use this method. This helps to make certain that justification for continued treatment is present in the note, and is a good method for setting up the plan. Following are some examples:

+ *Resident would benefit from environmental cues to orient him to the environment.*
+ *Consumer would benefit from continued instruction in problem-solving and anger management techniques needed for successful personal and social relationships.*

✦ *Client would benefit from further instruction in IADL tasks along with visual perceptual and problem-solving activities to increase safety.*

✦ *Veteran would benefit from activities that encourage trunk rotation to facilitate transfers and dressing skills.*

✦ *Consumer would benefit from continued mental health education including recognition of his delusions, need for medication, how it can help him, and why it is essential to his recovery.*

✦ *Client would benefit from instruction in use of reacher, sock-aide, and long-handled shoe horn to aid in LE dressing.*

✦ *Resident would benefit from skilled instruction in sequencing of tasks to increase safety while performing ADL tasks.*

✦ *Client would benefit from instruction in energy conservation techniques to perform meal preparation and clean-up.*

✦ *Child would benefit from continued use of modalities which ↓ tactile defensiveness as well as establishment of home program for parents to carry out with child.*

✦ *Infant would benefit from therapeutic exercises on therapy ball to encourage trunk extension needed for postural control during play activities.*

Make sure that you are **specific** with your description of what the client would benefit from and why it is important. A common mistake by students and new therapists when learning to write the "A" is making a vague statement that the client would benefit from more of the same techniques that have already been provided without specifying the targeted outcome.

Too vague:	*Client would benefit from continued ADL training.*
Better:	*Client would benefit from instruction in use of tub bench and hand-held shower to increase safety during bathing.*

Too vague:	*Student would benefit from continued visual perceptual activities.*
Better:	*Student would benefit from visual memory activities to improve ability to copy math problems from board to paper.*

When you justify the need for continued OT services, it is necessary to document the reason the service must be provided by an OT or OTA rather than by another professional or by nonprofessional personnel. The *Scope of Practice* (AOTA, 2010c) and *Guidelines for Supervision, Roles, and Responsibilities During the Delivery of Occupational Therapy Services* (AOTA, 2009) outline the services that require an OT practitioner.

OTs provide the following services:

✦ Evaluating clients, identifying problems, establishing goals, and developing intervention plans

✦ Reviewing the effectiveness of the intervention and modifying the intervention plan as needed

OTs *and* OTAs provide the following services:

✦ Modification of functional activities and/or instruction in compensatory techniques

✦ Instruction in the use of adaptive equipment for functional activities

✦ Health promotion and wellness activities to enhance occupational performance

✦ Training in ADLs, IADLs, and community/work reintegration

✦ Provision of individualized education to clients, family members, and caregivers

✦ Modification of environments to enhance occupational performance

✦ Fabrication of splints and other orthotic devices

✦ Training in use of prosthetic devices

✦ Training in assistive technology and adaptive devices

✦ Management of feeding and swallowing deficits

✦ Application of physical agent modalities to enhance occupational performance

✦ Management of wound care and use of manual therapy techniques

✦ Driver rehabilitation and community mobility

✦ Therapeutic exercises and activities to develop, remediate, or compensate for deficits in performance skills

Skilled OT is **not** evident when the OT or OTA provides the following services:

✦ Continuing treatment after goals are reached or no further significant progress is expected

✦ Carrying out a maintenance program

✦ Providing routine strengthening or exercise programs if there is no potential for functional improvement

✦ Carrying out daily programs after the adapted procedures are in place and no further progress is expected

✦ Presenting information in the form of handouts or videos without having the client or caregiver **perform** the activity (e.g., energy conservation techniques; donning of post-surgical corset)

✦ Providing services to a client who has poor rehabilitation potential

✦ Duplicating services with another discipline

Wording is critical to documenting the necessity for continued skilled OT. The OT practitioner **provides skilled instruction** to clients rather than **assisting** them. For example, an OT may provide instruction in methods of energy conservation and work simplification instead of helping the client perform a strenuous task. OTs **design** home programs and OTs or OTAs may provide **instruction** in home programs, which will then be carried out by clients, aides, or family members.

Why should a client's funding source reimburse you to watch a client carry out the home exercise program that he performs daily on his own? If you are **evaluating** his ability to do all the components of it correctly, or **modifying** it to compensate for recent progress, then your professional skill is clearly required. Analyze your clinical reasoning and then document the principles and strategies used during a treatment session in justifying the continuation of skilled OT services. Refer to Worksheet 9-2 for practice in determining which services would justify continued OT treatment.

Remember that the justification for continued treatment must support the frequency and duration of the plan that you will establish in the "P" section of your note. If the last sentence of your "A" reads, *"Client would benefit from information on energy conservation techniques,"* do not expect the payer to approve more than one more treatment session.

If this is your last session, complete the sentence with what the client would benefit from after discharge. For example:

✦ *Following discharge from rehab unit, client would benefit from home health OT to assess need for home adaptations to accommodate use of w/c for ADLs and IADLs.*

✦ *Client would benefit from continued PROM provided by restorative aide in order to prevent ® UE contracture and skin breakdown.*

✦ *Child would benefit from OT re-evaluation in 6 months to determine if fine motor skills are developing at an age-appropriate level.*

WRITING THE ASSESSMENT

As you read carefully through the material in your "S" and "O," it is sometimes helpful to make a quick list of things you want to discuss in the "A" section of your note. For example, consider "S" and "O":

S: *Client stated that he gets bored during the day when he has nothing to do, and said, "I wish I had a car so I could get out easier."*

O: *Client participated in 90-minute OT session in his home, on city bus, and at grocery store for community reintegration following discharge from inpatient facility. Client demonstrated home management skills and ability to care for pets by simulation. Client was able to identify which bus to catch to go to grocery store, but needed reassurance that his choice was correct. At the grocery store, client independently chose lunch meat and fruit for lunches this week, but needed SBA for payment.*

The therapist identified the following problems, progress, potential, and need for continued services:

Problems:

✦ Client is anxious about whether his bus choice is really correct.

✦ Client is still unable to manage money independently.

Progress:

✦ Client is able to simulate care of home and pets.

✦ Client is able to choose the correct bus to get to the grocery store.

✦ Client is willing to choose healthier foods at the store this visit.

Potential
+ In this therapist's professional judgment, the progress shown to date is also a good indicator of rehab potential for this client.

Need for Continued Services:
+ Client still needs to improve community mobility and money management skills in order to increase functional independence.

A: *Client's ability to demonstrate home and pet care activities as taught earlier shows good progress toward being able to live independently in the community. Client also demonstrates good progress in community mobility by being able to identify which bus to take to the grocery store this visit, and in ability to care for self by choosing healthier foods than his former choices of chips and donuts. Anxiety level in selecting the correct bus and need for assistance in managing money continue to limit client's functional independence. Client would benefit from continued instruction in going new places in the community and instruction in money management to increase his ability to shop without caregiver support.*

Here are a few more examples of what the completed assessment of a note might look like:

A: *Inability to don Ⓛ LE prosthesis Ⓘ currently limits Ⓘ in ambulation needed for functional toileting. Pt. demonstrates progress this session by requiring only min Ⓐ to don prosthesis as compared to mod Ⓐ required yesterday. Pt.'s recent progress and motivation are good indications of potential to be Ⓘ with management of prosthesis. Client would benefit from additional skilled instruction in use of pulley-like fasteners installed this date on prosthesis to allow one-handed closure.*

A: *Fear, isolation, and decreased activity tolerance limit Dominique's independent living skills and are the focus of current treatment. Emerging willingness to initiate conversation with others and to initiate daily bathing and grooming indicate good progress toward goals. She has good potential to return to the level of independence she had prior to her recent psychotic episode. Dominique would benefit from continued skilled instruction in self-care skills as well as increased socialization and physical activity in order to be successful with community re-entry.*

A: *Child's Ⓛ neglect continues to limit her independence in self-care and play tasks. Spontaneous use of Ⓛ hand as a functional assist 60% of the time demonstrates progress from less than 50% spontaneous use during prior visits. She would benefit from facilitation of more bilateral activities to ↑ use of Ⓛ hand during play, as well as establishment of a home program for foster parents to carry out in between bi-weekly visits.*

A: *Client's spontaneous actions in groups, willingness to share verbally, and improved dress and hygiene seem to indicate an improved mood this week. Progress also noted in unprompted attendance, which is up this week from 2/8 to 6/8 groups attended. Goals #1 (assertion) and #2 (communication) are met as of this date. Client is demonstrating excellent potential for successful community re-entry. Client continues to have difficulty identifying leisure activities, and Goal #3 (leisure skills) will be continued through discharge. Client would benefit from continued instruction and opportunities in formulating a plan for use of leisure time.*

Notice in the last example above that the problems, progress, and rehab potential do not have to be in a particular order. Sometimes it makes more sense to identify the progress first and then comment on the remaining problems that justify continued services. Let's walk through one more example in a step-by-step manner.

Mrs. W's Stroke

Molly W is a 62-year-old woman who had a stroke 3 weeks ago. She lives with her husband of 40 years in a one-story home. Her husband works full time as an account manager at a local bank. She has good return in her involved lower extremity and is getting some return in her UE as well. She intends to return home to live with her husband and will be alone during the day while he is at work. (You met Mrs. W in Chapter 7 when you chose a subjective statement for her treatment session.)

S: *Client says she has difficulty moving Ⓡ UE, although she does not know why it will not move. She reports, "It really doesn't hurt. It's just tight."*

O: *Client participated in 30-minute OT session in rehab gym for UE activities to ↑ AROM in Ⓡ shoulder, activity tolerance, UE strength, and dynamic standing balance, in order to ↑ independence in ADL tasks.*
ADLs: In room, client was instructed in safety techniques and adaptive equipment use in toileting. Client needs Ⓑ grab bars in bathroom for safe sit → stand transition during toileting. Client attempted to stand by pulling on walker and one grab bar. Client was educated on safety issues and the use of Ⓑ grab bars; she verbalized understanding of recommendations.

Performance Skills: Client required CGA for balance during sit ↔ stand. In order to address activity tolerance, dynamic standing balance, and ↑ AROM in Ⓡ shoulder, client moved canned goods from counter to cupboard for 5 minutes before needing a 2-minute seated rest break. After resting, she participated in activities to ↑ dynamic standing balance by pouring liquid from a pitcher while standing with CGA for balance. After a 1-minute seated rest, client continued activities to ↑ dynamic standing balance and safety by retrieving objects from floor using reacher while ambulating c̄ wheeled walker and CGA.
Client Factors: Ⓡ shoulder abduction AROM <90°. Ⓡ shoulder abduction PROM WFL.

How would you assess this information? What **problems** can you identify? Safety risks? Are there performance skills that are not WFL that OT might impact? Do you see evidence of **progress**? Is there any indication of the client's rehab **potential**? What would this client **benefit from**?

The therapist identified the following problems, progress, potential, and need for continued services:

Problems:

✦ Client is unsafe during toilet transfer.

✦ Client has ↓ AROM in Ⓡ shoulder, ↓ activity tolerance, and ↓ dynamic standing balance.

Progress:

✦ Client verbalized understanding of safety instructions

Potential:

✦ Ⓡ UE PROM is WNL

✦ In this therapist's professional judgment, the client has good potential to return home independently.

Need for Continued Services:

✦ Client needs to improve AROM, strength, and activity tolerance and also needs instruction in safety and energy conservation techniques.

In preparing an assessment of the data in this note, this therapist identified two main problem areas: the safety of transferring to/from the toilet, and the client factors that were not WFL. This therapist was particularly concerned about the safety issues and addressed those first. She also noted the rehabilitation potential that would be helpful to a reviewer in deciding whether the client's progress is sufficient to justify the expense of treatment.

A: *Impulsivity and ↓ dynamic standing balance pose safety concern during sit → stand transfer for toileting. Verbalization of understanding safety instructions demonstrates progress and indicates that the client has the potential to progress to independence.*

Next she addressed the clinical reasoning behind devoting time to addressing client factors, in the light of her rehab potential.

A: *Impulsivity and ↓ dynamic standing balance pose safety concern during sit → stand transfer for toileting. Verbalization of understanding safety instructions demonstrates progress and indicates that the client has the potential to progress to independence.* **Client's ↓ AROM in Ⓡ shoulder, ↓ activity tolerance, and ↓ dynamic standing balance all interfere with ability to complete ADL tasks safely and independently.**

She completes the assessment by justifying continued treatment.

A: *Impulsivity and ↓ dynamic standing balance pose safety concern during sit → stand transfer for toileting. Verbalization of understanding safety instructions demonstrates progress and indicates that the client has the potential to progress to independence. Client's ↓ AROM in Ⓡ shoulder, ↓ activity tolerance, and ↓ dynamic standing balance all interfere with ability to complete ADL tasks safely and independently.* **Client would benefit from Ⓡ UE AROM and strengthening exercises along with continued skilled instruction in safety issues and energy conservation techniques.**

In this case, the therapist decided that the client factors could be addressed in two different ways, both by working on ↑ AROM, strength, and activity tolerance, and by teaching some energy conservation techniques. We know that payment for ongoing treatment of range and strength is often denied. In Chapter 10, you will see how this therapist plans to provide the services this client would benefit from in a cost-effective manner.

WORKSHEET 9-1

Writing About Problems in the Assessment

You will be rewriting some statements to make them more effective assessment statements using the following formula:

Contributing Factor	Impact	Ability to Engage in Occupation

For example, this statement is an observation:

Client's activity tolerance for lower body dressing was <2 minutes secondary to SOB from COPD.

It tells you what the therapist observed while providing intervention. To make it into an assessment statement, you would need to change the emphasis by turning the statement around to make the contributing factors the **subject** of the sentence and by adding the impact that those factors have on her independence in dressing. Using the formula above, you might write:

Client's SOB and activity tolerance <2 minutes is insufficient to complete lower body dressing.

Rewrite the following statements using the formula given above.

1. *Client demonstrated difficulty with laundry and cooking tasks due to memory and sequencing deficits.*

2. *Decreased level of arousal noted during morning dressing activities, requiring redirection to task.*

3. *Client unable to follow hip precautions during morning dressing due to memory deficits.*

4. *Client problem solved poorly while performing lower body dressing, as evidenced by multiple attempts required to button pants and don socks successfully.*

WORKSHEET 9-2

Justifying Continued Treatment

Which of the following require the skills of an occupational therapist?

___ Evaluation of a client

___ The practice of coordination and self-care skills on a daily basis

___ Establishing measurable, behavioral, objective, and individualized goals

___ Developing intervention plans designed to meet established goals

___ Analyzing and modifying functional activities through the provision of adaptive equipment or techniques

___ Determining that the modified tasks are safe and effective

___ Carrying out a maintenance program

___ Teaching the client to use the breathing techniques he has learned while performing ADL activities

___ Providing individualized instruction to the client, family, or caregiver

___ Modifying the intervention plan based on a re-evaluation

___ Donning/doffing of a client's resting hand splint on a regular schedule throughout the day

___ Providing specialized instruction to eliminate limitations in a functional activity

___ Developing a home program and instructing caregivers

___ Making changes in the environment

___ Teaching compensatory skills

___ Gait training

___ Adding instruction in lower body dressing techniques to a current ADL program

___ Presenting informational handouts without having the client perform the activity

___ Teaching adaptive techniques such as one-handed shoe tying

___ Routine exercise and strengthening programs

Worksheet 9-3

Writing the Assessment—Ellie's Development

Ellie was born prematurely at 24 weeks gestation. She is currently almost 7 months old, with an adjusted age of 3 months. She was referred to OT while in the NICU for stimulation of normal developmental sequence and continues to receive OT services because she is considered a high-risk infant.

S: *Parent reports that infant is gaining ~1 oz per day and will probably be able to discontinue O_2 "in a couple days."*

O: *Infant participated in 30-minute OT session in home to assess visual skills and to ↑ mobility skills related to play (head righting, rolling supine → side lying, and push-up in prone). Infant oriented to black & white illuminated design by turning head. Infant demonstrated visual tracking in horizontal plane 20° past midline. Infant unable to roll, right head, or push up in prone (Ⓘ), but with facilitation of weight shift and proximal stability, infant could perform activities after about 20 seconds and hold position. Infant became fatigued and "fussy" after 20 minutes of treatment, with four 1-minute rest breaks.*

How would you assess this information? What problems can you identify? Are there any contributing factors that OT might impact? What influence do the limiting factors above have on Ellie's ability to engage in occupation that is appropriate for her age? Do you see evidence of progress? Is there any indication of Ellie's rehab potential? What would she benefit from?

The therapist who is working with Ellie was concerned about the following:

✦ Inability to perform age-appropriate mobility skills Ⓘ during play

✦ Became fatigued after 20 minutes

✦ Lack of head righting responses

✦ Needs O_2

She was encouraged by the following:

✦ Need for O_2 is decreasing and she is gaining weight

✦ Ability to hold position if facilitated

✦ Ability to orient to a black and white image and to visually track horizontally

Write an assessment to add to the "S" and "O" given above.

A:

WORKSHEET 9-4

Writing the Assessment—Ms. D's Social Skills

Ms. D is a 35-year-old woman who has a diagnosis of bipolar disorder, although in a prior admission, she was diagnosed with schizophrenia. One of her goals is to talk to the mental health center staff about her problems rather than acting out her feelings. Today she was seen in social skills group with five other clients who also need help with relationship issues.

S: *Client reports that she understands the purpose of social skills group. She expressed a desire to attend all of the groups, saying that they are "fun."*

O: *Client participated in 60-minute social skills group focusing on friendship. Client appeared unkempt, with hair not combed and shirt rumpled. Client engaged in conversation with the other clients and the facilitator. Client interrupted others on 5 occasions. Client spontaneously verbalized her experiences with past friendships and her ideas of useful ways to make new friendships, but had to be redirected to the topic twice during discussion.*

1. What problems do you see in the above "S" and "O"?

2. What areas of occupation do these problems impact?

3. What evidence of progress and/or potential do you see?

4. What would this client benefit from?

5. Write a complete assessment statement for this note.

A:

Chapter 10

Writing the "P"—Plan

The last section of a SOAP note is the **plan**. In this section, you document the anticipated frequency and duration of your services and the specific interventions that will be used to achieve the client's goals. The plan should relate to the information presented in the "O" and the "A" and should address your assessment of what the client would benefit from. The "P" will inform your reader of your priorities regarding intervention strategies.

> Note: In an initial evaluation report, the "P" section will also contain the long-term and short-term goals. This will be covered in Chapter 12 when you learn more about intervention planning.

In some settings, you will see the "P" simply written as *"Continue plan of care."* For purposes of learning in this manual, that is NOT a sufficient plan. Your "P" should include:

- Frequency (how often; may also include length of session in some settings)
  - *Infant will be seen **2x/wk.**...*
  - *Continue OT **daily**...*
  - *Client will be seen **30 minutes b.i.d.**...*
- Duration (how long OT will continue)
  - *Infant will be seen 2x/wk. for **2 months**...*
  - *Continue OT daily for **3 days**...*
  - *Client will be seen 30 minutes b.i.d. for **1 week**...*
- Purpose of continued therapy and/or specific interventions
  - *Infant will be seen 2x/wk. for 2 months **to address feeding skills. Treatment to include oral desensitization and caregiver training in use of adaptive bottles.***
  - *Continue OT daily for 3 days **for skilled instruction in ADLs and IADLs. Sessions will focus on education in post-surgical hip precautions and adaptive equipment to maximize safety and independence in preparation for return to independent living situation.***
  - *Client will be seen 30 minutes b.i.d. for 1 week **to address visual perceptual and cognitive skills necessary for safe performance of ADLs and IADLs. Environmental modifications will be made to improve visual scanning to Ⓛ side during basic ADLs. Telephone book activity planned for afternoon session tomorrow.***

In each of the above examples, another therapist could read your "P" and know exactly how to proceed with this client's treatment. Consider some of the situations in which this would be crucial to providing quality care for your client:

Gateley CA, Borcherding S. *Documentation Manual for Occupational Therapy: Writing SOAP Notes, 3rd Edition* (pp. 105-112)
© 2012 SLACK Incorporated

✦ In acute care and rehabilitation settings, treatment may be provided 7 days per week and the client will encounter multiple occupational therapists during his or her hospital stay. Writing a thorough "P" ensures that the next therapist to see the client will use the client's therapy time efficiently to work toward meeting goals.

✦ In any setting where an OTA will be providing services, a thorough "P" is critical for communication between the OT and the OTA.

✦ Unexpected therapist absences happen in any setting. The "P" section of your note should allow another therapist to continue the client's treatment without interruption.

Here are some more examples of a "P":

✦ *Resident to be seen for 2 more weeks for ½-hr b.i.d. sessions for skilled instruction in meal preparation and clean-up. Focus will be on independent use of microwave using wheeled walker for mobility.*

✦ *Child will continue to be seen 1x/wk. for 30-minute sessions until IEP review in order to ↑ fine motor skills for better classroom performance. OT sessions to address handwriting and cutting skills.*

✦ *Client will continue to be seen in groups 5x/wk. for 1 week to work on social participation. Group sessions to address assertion skills and anger management techniques.*

✦ *Consumer will continue sheltered workshop program 5 days/wk. for 1 month to ↑ work skills. Target behaviors are improved attention to task and ability to follow 2-step directions.*

✦ *Continue 1 hr. daily sessions for 1 week for skilled ADL training. One-handed dressing techniques for donning shirt will be taught and button hook will be introduced.*

You must use your clinical judgment when determining frequency and duration of services. In many cases, there are expected norms of frequency and duration based on setting, funding source, or physician's order. For example:

✦ In a school setting, the frequency of services will be determined in the child's annual IEP meeting and will remain the same until the IEP is modified.

✦ In an acute care setting, patients who have had orthopedic surgery likely will have OT services once or twice daily for the duration of the hospital stay, but this may vary depending on each surgeon's protocol for therapy services.

✦ Patients who are admitted to a hospital for general medical issues such as pneumonia or other illness often have only one or two OT sessions to assess ability to return home.

✦ Patients in an inpatient rehabilitation facility typically have OT for 60 or 90 minutes daily (generally split between 2 sessions), depending on the amount of physical therapy and speech therapy services that they are receiving.

✦ Residents of long-term care facilities may receive OT services a few times a week to daily depending on the individual situation and client needs.

✦ Home health clients may have just a few OT visits to assess home safety or may continue OT services a few times a week for several weeks to address functional deficits.

✦ Clients in an inpatient psychiatric setting may have both individual and group sessions on a daily basis during their stay.

✦ In an outpatient setting, a physician may write orders that specify the frequency and duration of OT services.

✦ Early intervention services typically range from monthly consultation to direct services 1 or more times weekly.

✦ Funding sources may dictate the number of OT visits that will be paid, such as 60 minutes weekly for 8 weeks.

Please note that the above examples are not standards. They are simply provided to demonstrate that the frequency and duration of services will vary greatly among settings and situations. You must be familiar with the expectations of your particular setting.

COMPLETING THE PLAN FOR MRS. W

Now let us write a plan for the note on Mrs. W that we assessed in the last chapter. As you recall from Chapter 9, Mrs. W is a 62-year-old woman who had a stroke 3 weeks ago. She has good return in her involved LE and is getting some return in her UE as well. She intends to return home to live with her husband and will be alone during the day while he is at work.

S: *Client says she has difficulty moving* ⓇUE, *although she does not know why it will not move. She reports, "It really doesn't hurt. It's just tight."*

O: *Client participated in 30-minute OT session in rehab gym for UE activities to ↑ AROM in* Ⓡ *shoulder, activity tolerance, UE strength, and dynamic standing balance in order to ↑ independence in ADL tasks.*

ADLs: In room, client was instructed in safety techniques and adaptive equipment use in toileting. Client needs Ⓑ *grab bars in bathroom for safe sit → stand transition during toileting. Client attempted to stand by pulling on walker and one grab bar. Client was educated on safety issues and the use of* Ⓑ *grab bars; she verbalized understanding of recommendations.*

Performance Skills: Client required CGA for balance during sit ↔ stand. In order to address activity tolerance, dynamic standing balance, and ↑ AROM in Ⓡ *shoulder, client moved canned goods from counter to cupboard for 5 minutes before needing a 2-minute seated rest break. After resting, she participated in activities to ↑ dynamic standing balance by pouring liquid from a pitcher while standing with CGA for balance. After a 1-minute seated rest, client continued activities to ↑ dynamic standing balance and safety by retrieving objects from floor using reacher while ambulating c̄ wheeled walker and CGA.*

Client Factors: Ⓡ *shoulder abduction AROM <90°.* Ⓡ *shoulder abduction PROM WFL.*

A: *Impulsivity and ↓ dynamic standing balance pose safety concern during sit → stand transfer for toileting. Verbalization of understanding safety instructions demonstrates progress and indicates that the client has the potential to progress to independence. Client's ↓ AROM in* Ⓡ *shoulder, ↓ activity tolerance, and ↓ dynamic standing balance all interfere with ability to complete ADL tasks safely and independently. Client would benefit from* Ⓡ *UE AROM and strengthening exercises along with continued skilled instruction in safety issues and energy conservation techniques.*

In the "A" above, the therapist has already justified the main things she intends to do and indicated the client's rehabilitation potential. Now she needs to be specific about how often the client will be treated and for what length of time. She first specifies the frequency and duration of treatment:

P: ***Continue to treat client 5x/wk. for 1 week*** . . .

She could have specified the length of the treatment sessions (e.g., "*for 1 hr. sessions*"), but this therapist chose not to do that in this particular note. Next she specifies how she plans to use the treatment time:

P: *Continue to treat client 5x/wk. for 1 week **for skilled instruction in safe transfers and toileting**. . .*

Since she anticipates discharge in 1 week, she has to prioritize her time. She chooses to work on balance and energy conservation as a part of functional mobility during ADL activities. Since she has already written in the "A" that the client would benefit from additional AROM and strengthening exercises, she now needs to specify how she plans to address this need as well:

P: *Continue to treat client 5x/wk. for 1 week for skilled instruction in safe transfers and toileting. **Plan to address dynamic standing balance and to provide skilled instruction in energy conservation techniques. Home program for AROM and strengthening exercises for** Ⓡ **shoulder will be taught.***

This note is now complete. This therapist has demonstrated clinical reasoning in planning for discharge in advance of the discharge date. In later notes, she will indicate the client's progress in learning the home program, since simply handing the client a set of printed exercises is not considered a skilled or billable service. The client's progress in learning the home program will also confirm that the therapist's assessment of the client's rehabilitation potential was on target.

WORKSHEET 10-1

Completing the Plan for Ellie

In the last chapter, you wrote an assessment for a treatment note on Ellie's development. Now you will complete that note by adding a plan. As you recall from Chapter 9, Ellie is a 7-month-old infant (adjusted age of 3 months following premature birth at 24 weeks gestation). She was seen in the NICU and continues to receive OT services because she is considered a high-risk infant.

In the last sentence of your "A," you have established what you want to do. In your "P," state how often you plan to see Ellie, how long each session will last, how long you plan to continue your intervention before re-evaluating or discontinuing treatment, and how you plan to use your time.

S: *Parent reports that infant is gaining ~1 oz per day and will probably be able to discontinue O_2 "in a couple days."*

O: *Infant participated in 30-minute OT session in home to assess visual skills and to ↑ mobility skills related to play (head righting, rolling supine → side lying, and push-up in prone). Infant oriented to black & white illuminated design by turning head. Infant demonstrated visual tracking in horizontal plane 20° past midline. Infant unable to roll, right head, or push up in prone Ⓘ, but with facilitation of weight shift and proximal stability, infant could perform activities after about 20 seconds and hold position. Infant became fatigued and "fussy" after 20 minutes of treatment, with four 1-minute rest breaks.*

A: *Decreased postural control and need for facilitation of weight shift limits infant's ability to perform early mobility skills needed for play. Limited mobility combined with her tolerance for less than 20 minutes of activity and the need for frequent rest breaks limit her ability to explore her environment and reach developmental milestones at a typical age. Ability to perform transitional movements with facilitation, orientation to black and white design, and ability to track in horizontal plane show good potential for future developmental gains. Infant would benefit from continued OT services to stimulate developmental skills and from parent education in a home program.*

P:

WORKSHEET 10-2

Completing the Plan for Ms. D

As you recall from Chapter 9, Ms. D is a 35-year-old woman who has a diagnosis of bipolar disorder, although in a prior admission, she was diagnosed with schizophrenia. One of her goals is to talk to the mental health center staff about her problems rather than acting out her feelings. Today she was seen in social skills group with five other clients who also need help with relationship issues.

You have noted in the last sentence of your assessment some of the areas of intervention that you think might benefit Ms. D. Now you will fill in the specifics of your plan.

S: *Client reports that she understands the purpose of social skills group. She expressed a desire to attend all of the groups, saying that they are "fun."*

O: *Client participated in 60-minute social skills group focusing on friendship. Client appeared unkempt, with hair not combed and shirt rumpled. Client engaged in conversation with the other clients and the facilitator. Client interrupted others on 5 occasions. Client spontaneously verbalized her experiences with past friendships and her ideas of useful ways to make new friendships, but had to be redirected to the topic twice during discussion.*

A: *Client's unkempt appearance, interrupting behaviors, and need for redirection to topic of conversation interfere with her ability to engage in social participation with peers. Her expressed interest in groups and her willingness to engage in conversation and share her ideas show good potential to develop relationships and to express herself verbally in place of acting out. Client would benefit from participating in groups where conversational skills are stressed, from further facilitation of attention to social cues, and from instruction in ADL activities stressing hygiene and appearance.*

P:

11

Making Good Notes Even Better

Now that you have learned to write effective SOAP notes, it is time to review your work and take your skills to the next level. We will begin by reviewing problem statements and goals, and then we will review each of the SOAP categories. As we review, you will have an opportunity to refine your skills beyond the basics learned so far by completing the worksheets at the end of this chapter.

Problem Statements

As you recall, a problem list is developed from your initial assessment. Problems are defined as areas of occupation that are not within functional limits (WFL) and that you plan to address through OT intervention. Problem statements need both a **contributing factor** (client factor, performance skill, contextual limitation, etc.) and a related **area of occupation**. Remember that the best problem statements also give a way of measuring the extent of the problem (such as "*needs mod assist*"). Also remember that those clients who use our services are more than an assist level, and we make a statement in terms of what the client is **unable to do** or **needs assistance in doing** rather than saying that the client **is** a particular assist level.

Writing Measurable Occupation-Based Goals and Objectives

You have a method for writing goals that will ensure that all the necessary components are present:
+ C–Client   Client will perform
+ O–Occupation   What occupation?
+ A–Assist Level   With what level of assistance/independence?
+ S–Specific Condition Under what conditions?
+ T–Timeline   By when?

Remember that sometimes the order of the elements must be rearranged so that your goal statement does not sound awkward. Another tip you learned about writing observations is to de-emphasize the treatment media. That is also important in goal writing. Consider the following goal:

Client will place 8 half-inch screws and washers on a block of wood with holes by the next treatment session.

This goal emphasizes the treatment media and is not occupation-based. Written in a different way, the targeted occupation of work becomes evident and the treatment media becomes the **specific condition** rather than the focus of the goal:

By the end of the 2nd treatment session, client will complete work simulation task by placing 8 half-inch screws into a block of wood in <5 minutes.

Gateley CA, Borcherding S. *Documentation Manual for Occupational Therapy: Writing SOAP Notes, 3rd Edition* (pp. 113-142)
© 2012 SLACK Incorporated

The SOAP Structure

"S"—Subjective

In this section, you report anything significant that the client says about his or her treatment. If the client is unable to speak, report on his or her nonverbal communication, if any. In the case of a young child, a confused client, or a client who is unable to communicate, you may use what the primary caregiver says.

"O"—Objective

Writing Good Opening Lines

This section begins with an opening line that explains where the session took place, for how long, and the purpose of the session. It is essential that you indicate that the client and/or caregiver was an active participant and that you show your professional skill as an OT in the first sentence of the "O." For example, suppose you are treating a client whose contractures are compromising his positioning. Instead of saying, *"Client seen for positioning,"* you might introduce your "O" by saying one of the following:

- *Caregivers participated in 15-minute bedside OT session for education on positioning client to prevent skin breakdown.*
- *Pt. participated in 30-minute session in home to select positioning strategies to improve seated posture for mealtimes.*

In another scenario, suppose your client is ambulating as a part of IADL activities. Since this might potentially be seen as a duplication of services with PT, you would need to be careful about the words you use. Instead of saying, *"Client seen for ambulation,"* you might say:

Client participated in 30-minute IADL session in rehab kitchen to increase dynamic standing balance and attention to Ⓛ UE for safety when ambulating around kitchen to prepare meals.

Being Specific About Assist Levels

Remember that you also need to be specific about **the part of the task** that required assistance, rather than reporting only the level of assistance needed.

Not specific enough: *Client supine → sit max Ⓐ, sit → stand mod Ⓐ.*

Specific: *Client supine → sit with max Ⓐ to lift body weight, sit → stand with mod Ⓐ for balance and to maintain TTWB precautions.*

There is a difference between telling **why** the assist was needed, for example:

*Client needed mod Ⓐ to transfer w/c → bed **due to flaccid left side**.*

and **the part of the task** that required assistance, for example:

*Client needed mod Ⓐ **to stand and pivot** when transferring w/c → bed.*

When writing about assist levels in your "O," please specify **what part of the task** required assistance.

Writing a Complete and Concise "O"

In the objective section of the note, you report what you observed while providing treatment for the client, either chronologically or in categories. As you gain skill in documentation, you become more aware of what to include and what to omit in order to be concise. Below is an observation that is very concise. Read it and spend a few minutes deciding what it needs to make it better before reading on.

> **O**:   *Client participated in 60-minute session in room for ADLs and transfer training.*
> *ADLs: Client donned robe with set-up. Client donned/doffed socks with set-up.*
> *Mobility: Bed → chair with CGA; supine → sit Ⓘ.*

This note does not have enough information. It is **too** concise. There needs to be some indication that skilled OT was provided. You could start with an opening statement that shows why your skill as an OT is needed in this situation. As it stands, it is apparent that someone observed the client dress and transfer and recorded assist levels, but a rehabilitation aide or nursing staff could have done this.

Second, the time required to do the activities documented in this note could be very short. If this is a 1-hour treatment session, what else was done? If the client was slow to do the things recorded above, what caused so few activities to take so long? Is there a cognitive problem? Is there a coordination, safety, or motor planning problem? Were adapted techniques or adaptive equipment used to allow the client to be independent?

Third, with this client's documented level of independence, there is nothing in this note to justify further skilled OT. Unless this is the client's last session, information needs to be provided that will justify continued treatment.

"A"—ASSESSMENT

This is your professional opinion about the meaning of what you have just observed. In assessing your data, you will pay special attention to evidence of problems, progress, and rehab potential. The assessment ends with a statement of what the client would benefit from.

Writing Effective Assessment Statements

When OTs are first beginning to write SOAP notes, it is sometimes difficult to decide what is an observation and what is an assessment. Anything you see a client do is an observation. Its **meaning** in terms of your client's ability to function in some area of occupation is your assessment. Sometimes the difference between an observation and an assessment is one of emphasis. Remember the formula that puts the contributing factor as the subject of your sentence:

Contributing Factor	Impact	Ability to Engage in Occupation

+ Identify the contributing factor (e.g., ↓ *AROM*; *inability to sequence*; or *narrow doorways*) and make it the subject of your sentence to give it the emphasis it needs in this section of your note.
+ Decide whether the area of difficulty you observed today is an indicator of a broader area of occupation. For example, is the decreased AROM you observed during grooming also a problem in other ADL tasks? Will the client's inability to balance a checkbook also cause problems with other money management tasks? Do the problems you observed today put his or her safety at risk?
+ Make certain your assessment statement tells how the problem areas impact the client's ability to engage in meaningful occupation. After each problem you note (e.g., limited AROM, sequencing deficits, unstable balance), ask yourself "So what?" So he or she is unstable to do that–what difference does that make? The answer to your "So what?" question is your assessment of the situation.

Let's consider some examples of how an observation statement would be worded differently than an assessment statement. For example, suppose you are working with a client who tells you she plans to return home to live alone in her farmhouse. You have worked on teaching her some energy conservation techniques, but she forgets to incorporate those into her morning dressing routine. What is the basic or core problem for this client? Why does it matter? The following statement is an **observation** of the client's behavior:

> *Pt. was unable to use energy conservation techniques during morning dressing due to memory deficit.*

However, phrased differently, it becomes an **assessment** of what was observed:

> *Memory deficit interferes with client's ability to retain instructions in compensatory techniques such as energy conservation, which limits her ability to safely perform self-care tasks needed to return to prior* Ⓘ *living situation.*

Note that in this assessment statement, the OT has identified the basic or core problem as the client's inability to retain instructions she has been given. This might be followed by a recommendation to use memory cues of some kind. Otherwise, why should a payer continue to pay for instruction that will not be remembered? You might also want to consider her safety in living alone if her short-term memory is impaired.

According to the formula, the assessment does not repeat what was observed. Instead it begins with the contributing factor that is a problem, broadens the scope of the performance area to include related tasks, and answers the question "So what? Why does this matter in this client's life?" Let's look at another example. The following is an **observation** of what the OT saw today:

> *Client's problem solving was functional and accurate with verbal prompts.*

An **assessment** of this situation would sound like this:

Client's need for multiple verbal prompts to solve social problems limits his ability to respond appropriately in unstructured social situations and to enter into successful relationships with others. Ability to problem solve with verbal prompting indicates good potential to reach stated goals.

Note that in the observation statement, there was no area of occupation mentioned. In the assessment statement, the OT addressed the areas of occupation that are impacted by the client's ↓ problem-solving skills.

Let's look at one last example. The statement is an **observation** because it tells what the client did:

Client tolerated vestibular and proprioceptive input well today as evidenced by him choosing the activity.

Yes, the client choosing the activity is an indication of his tolerance, and that is good clinical reasoning, but there are more important things to **assess**. One is his progress in tolerating input, and the other is the impact that this progress has on his ability to engage in occupation

Client's choices of activities with proprioceptive and vestibular components indicate progress in sensory tolerance necessary for attention to task in the classroom.

Sweeping Assessment Statements

In the face of a busy schedule and serious time constraints, it is tempting to make concise and sweeping assessment statements, such as:

A: *Poor postural stability interferes with ADL performance. Improvement since last note shows good rehab potential. Client would benefit from continued activities to increase postural stability and ability to do personal ADL tasks.*

A: *Decreased strength and coordination prevent client from completing ADLs Ⓘ. Client's ability to follow instructions shows good rehab potential. Client would benefit from continued activities to increase strength, coordination, and fine motor skills.*

A: *Deficits in upper body strength, fine motor, and feeding limit Jordan's ability to be Ⓘ in home and classroom activities.*

While these are accurate, they are limited and would benefit from some elaboration. An elaboration on Jordan's note might read:

A: *Deficits in upper body strength limit Jordan's ability to be Ⓘ in eating and dressing. Decreased fine motor skills impede typical classroom activities such as holding a pencil or crayon and manipulating small items, as well as emerging IADL tasks in which Jordan is beginning to show interest. Jordan would benefit from continued upper body strengthening, reach-grasp-release activities, and feeding activities in order to reach developmental milestones more expediently.*

Here are two more examples of thorough assessments:

A: *Decreased cheek and lip range diminishes pressure in mouth needed for swallow, which results in inadequate swallow reflex. Poor suck and swallow pattern due to decreased oral musculature may lead to inadequate nutritional intake. Decreased head control with upright posture indicates poor head-righting skills, which will hinder Hannah during feeding. Demonstration of visual tracking in different planes indicates good rehab potential. Hannah would benefit from continued skilled OT for oral motor stretches, increased head control, increased oral motor skills, and a home program for prone position activities.*

A: *Ability to complete simple to complex bilateral eye coordination and visual scanning tasks in static position without verbal cues demonstrates improvements since last session. Eye coordination and visual scanning deficits during dynamic movement pose safety concern during functional mobility for IADLs. Ability to perform Ⓛ shoulder AROM with ↓ pain indicates improvement since last session. Client would benefit from further skilled OT in complex bilateral eye coordination and visual scanning activities during dynamic movement, and increased AROM in Ⓛ shoulder without pain in order to increase functional performance during ADL and IADL tasks.*

"P"—PLAN

Your plan contains a statement of the frequency, duration, and purpose of future OT visits for your client. Good plans also include a description of the intervention strategies that will address the client's goals.

Too concise: *Continue plan of care.*

Thorough: *Pt. will be seen for one more OT visit prior to discharge home to focus on safe ADL and IADL transfers. Client and spouse will be instructed in use of tub transfer bench and pt. will practice car transfers in simulated car in rehab gym.*

A COMPLETE SOAP NOTE

Let's look at a complete SOAP note that meets the criteria described in the last several sections.

S: *Client reported that she bent to the floor to pick up her makeup case this morning. She stated, "I just have a hard time remembering not to bend down." Daughter reports she will provide increased supervision to help client remember to follow hip precautions.*

O: *Client participated in 45-minute session in dining room with daughter present for skilled instruction in maintaining hip precautions during household management tasks. Client ambulated to dining room SBA for balance using wheeled walker. Client retrieved snack from refrigerator and utensils from drawer c̄ SBA for safety. Client required 4 verbal cues to remember hip precautions for stand → sit and when turning with walker. Following skilled instruction, client able to retrieve items from floor using a reacher. Education provided to client and daughter on hip precautions and safety during both basic and instrumental ADL tasks. Client and daughter both voiced understanding.*

A: *Client's inability to remember hip precautions during household management tasks without verbal cues puts her at risk for re-injury. Supportive daughter and ability to use adaptive equipment properly after instruction indicate good potential for reaching stated goals. Client would benefit from further skilled instruction in maintaining hip precautions during ADL tasks, sit ↔ stand, and transitional living skills.*

P: *Continue tx. 3x/wk. for 1 wk. to work on incorporating hip precautions into ADL and IADL tasks. Instruction of reacher will be continued, and written reminders (text & pictures) will be posted in prominent locations, including bathroom, bedroom, and kitchen.*

REVISING NOTES

The following note will help you apply the principles described earlier in this chapter. Jenna is a preschool child who is receiving OT twice weekly to increase her tolerance for sensory input. As you read each section of the note, consider what it needs to make it better.

"S"—SUBJECTIVE

S: *Grandma came in and stated, "Jenna was excited this morning to come see you girls." She also commented that Jenna tolerated a few seconds of tooth brushing this morning. Throughout session, Jenna stated several times, "wipe my hands" or "wipe my arms" when foam got on them for too long. She also cried out and yelled "stop" when she had enough of the oral ranging exercise.*

Revisions:
+ The first sentence is irrelevant unless the child usually resists attending.
+ The fact that the grandmother came in is irrelevant since we have her report.
+ The "S" could be much more concise yet still effective.

S: *Grandmother reports that Jenna now tolerates a few seconds of tooth brushing. Jenna asked for hands/arms to be wiped off and asked for oral ranging exercises to be stopped when her tolerance had been reached.*

"O"—Objective

O: *Child was seen in the clinic to decrease oral defensiveness.*
      Proprioception/Deep Pressure: *The therapist began the session with a variety of proprioception and deep pressure activities to allow Jenna to have a better sense of her position in space. Jenna chose to bounce on the big therapy ball first, needing CGA. Jenna then began jumping and sliding, which added a vestibular element. These activities prepped her to engage attentively to the remainder of the session.*
      Sensory: *The therapist presented Jenna with foam, water, and foam stick-ups to play with. Jenna was hesitant to play with or touch any of the objects, but after prompting Jenna actually touched the foam but immediately wanted her hands wiped off. Touching this texture is the beginning of a desensitization process that will assist her to be more tolerant of different textures for the purpose of feeding and hygiene.*
      Oral Motor: *The therapist introduced the idea of Jenna feeding the babies food in hopes of imitation. However, when Jenna put the spoon to her own moth, she began spitting. The therapist followed up this activity with completing oral resistive exercises of elongating and protruding the lips as well as stretching the cheek muscles. The intention is to increase length and range for speech and feeding. Jenna had an adverse reaction to this.*

Revisions:

✦ Opening statement needs to indicate active client participation and needs to specify duration and purpose of session.

✦ Delete what the therapist did and reword to focus on the client.

✦ De-emphasize the treatment media in the first category and talk about the purpose. Keep this brief, since it is only prep for the sensory and oral-motor work, or make it part of the introduction.

✦ In the opening statement, talk about sensory as well as oral motor.

✦ Make the note more concise.

✦ Avoid mixing "A" material into the observation.

✦ When talking about desensitizing, tell how much the client could tolerate, in order to measure progress.

O: *Child participated in 45-minute session in clinic to decrease oral and sensory defensiveness in preparation for accepting a wider range of textures during feeding and hygiene activities. Child tolerated 10 minutes of proprioception/deep pressure and vestibular input in preparation for engaging her attention in the therapy activities.*
      Sensory: *Child presented with foam, water, and foam stick-ups to desensitize her to textures used in feeding/hygiene, but was hesitant to touch any of the objects. After prompting, child touched the foam but immediately wanted it wiped off.*
      Oral Motor: *Child fed a baby doll as an intro to self-feeding. When putting the spoon to her own mouth, child began spitting. Child tolerated 45 seconds of oral resistive activities used to elongate and protrude the lips and stretch the cheek muscles for speech and feeding.*

"A"—Assessment

A: *Child has increased tolerance for proprioception activities, which has led to an increased ability for her to concentrate on one activity at a time. However, her unwillingness to engage in sensory activities with wet and semi-wet media is still a concern in relation to eating. Hopefully with continued desensitization and oral resistive exercise, Jenna will have decreased oral/tactile defensiveness.*

Revisions:

✦ We do not see any indication of ability to concentrate on one activity at a time. This is not a problem with the "A," but a change that would need to be made in the "O" so that we can assess it in the "A."

✦ The second sentence is good with a little revision. It is a sweeping assessment statement and covers a lot of material. Is there more that could be said about the session than this? Are there any other problems? What about the problems tolerating the oral resistive exercises? Is there any progress?

✦ The third sentence needs to be changed to what she would benefit from rather than what the therapist hopes.

A: *Increased tolerance (from 8 to 10 minutes) of proprioceptive activities has resulted in an increased ability to concentrate on one activity at a time. Ability to tolerate 45 seconds of oral resistive activities, willingness to bring spoon to her mouth, and tolerance for a few seconds of tooth brushing also indicate progress. Child's reluctance to engage in sensory activities with wet or semi-wet media continues to interfere with eating and hygiene. Client would benefit from continued desensitization and oral resistive exercises to decrease tactile defensiveness.*

"P"—Plan

P: *Continue plan of care.*

Revisions:
+ There is no mention of frequency, duration, or purpose.
+ There is no evidence of clinical reasoning that upcoming sessions will address issues that continue to limit this child's functional performance.

P: *Child will continue to be seen for 30-minute sessions 2x/wk for 3 months to increase tolerance of certain sensory media and to decrease oral defensiveness. Focus will be on increasing tolerated food textures and improving oral range needed for self-feeding. Grandmother will be instructed in home activities to enhance Jenna's development of sensory processing skills.*

The page that follows is a summary of everything you have learned about writing SOAP notes in occupational therapy. A copy of this page is provided at the back of this manual in a cardstock pullout. Pull it out and carry it with you to use as a quick-reference guide.

A Quick Checklist for Evaluating Your Note

Use the following summary chart as a quick-reference guide to be sure that your note contains all of the essential elements.

☐	**S:** Use something significant that the client says about his or her treatment or condition.
☐	**O:** Begin with a statement about the length, setting, and purpose of the treatment session, using wording that indicates active participation by the client.
☐	Follow the opening statement with a summary of what you have observed, either chronologically or using categories.
☐	Be professional, concise, and specific.
☐	Focus on occupation.
☐	Focus on the client's response to the treatment provided, rather than on what the therapist did.
☐	Write from the client's point of view, leaving yourself out.
☐	Be specific about assist levels.
☐	Avoid making a list of actions and assist levels.
☐	De-emphasize the treatment media.
☐	Make certain that it is clear that you were not just a passive observer in the session.
☐	Avoid judging the client.
☐	Use only standard abbreviations.
☐	**A:** Go sentence by sentence through the information presented in the "S" and the "O," asking yourself what it means for the client's ability to engage in meaningful occupation. Note what **problems**, **progress**, and **potential** for rehabilitation you see.
☐	Remember the formula that puts the contributing factor as the subject of your sentence: <table><tr><td>Contributing Factor</td><td>Impact</td><td>Ability to Engage in Occupation</td></tr></table>
☐	End the "A" with "*Client would benefit from…,*" justifying continued skilled OT and setting up the plan.
☐	Be sure that the time lines and activities you are putting in your plan match the skilled OT you say your client needs.
☐	**P:** Specify the frequency and duration of future OT sessions (e.g., 2x/wk for 4 wks).
☐	Describe the purpose of future OT sessions.
☐	Include a brief description of the intervention strategies that will address the client's goals.

If you have read the text carefully, you will know what each item means. For a more complete explanation, refer to the chapter that provides information in detail.

S:

✦ Use something significant that the client says about his or her treatment or condition. If there is nothing significant, ask yourself whether you are using your interview skills effectively to elicit the information about the client's perspective.

O:

✦ Begin with a statement about the length, setting, and purpose of the treatment session, using wording that indicates active participation by the client.

Client participated in 45-minute OT session in rehab kitchen for meal preparation activity.

✦ Focus on the client's response, rather than on what you did.

Client able to don socks using sock-aid after demonstration.

✦ Write from the client's point of view, leaving yourself out.

Client repositioned rather than *Therapist repositioned client.*

✦ Be specific about assist levels.

Client required min Ⓐ for hand placement during pivot transfer to toilet.

✦ De-emphasize the treatment media.

Client worked on tripod pinch using pegs in order to grasp objects needed for ADLs.

✦ Make certain that it is clear that you were not just a passive observer in the session. Don't just make a list of all the assist levels and think that is enough.

✦ Avoid judging the client. For example, say he *"…didn't complete the activity."* Don't add *"…because he was stubborn."*

A:

✦ Go sentence by sentence through the information presented in the "S" and the "O," asking yourself what it means for the client's ability to engage in meaningful occupation. Note what **problems**, **progress**, and **potential** for rehabilitation you see.

✦ Remember the formula that puts the contributing factor as the subject of your sentence:

Contributing Factor	Impact	Ability to Engage in Occupation

Deficits in UE AROM & strength limit client's ability to complete basic self-care tasks.

✦ End the "A" with *"Client would benefit from…,"* justifying continued skilled OT and setting up the plan.

Client would benefit from skilled instruction in energy conservation techniques, continued strengthening of UE, and compensatory techniques for performing IADLs one-handed.

P:

✦ Specify frequency, duration, and purpose of future sessions, and give a brief description of planned interventions.

Infant will be seen 2x/wk. for 2 months to address feeding skills. Treatment to include oral desensitization and caregiver training in use of adaptive bottles.

WORKSHEET 11-1

Writing Problem Statements

Consider the following problem statements. Decide what is needed to make each one a better problem statement, then rewrite the sentence into a better format.

1. *Pt unable to dress LE ① due to trunk instability.*

2. *Child doesn't tolerate very much classroom activity due to ↓ activity tolerance.*

3. *Consumer acts out.*

WORKSHEET 11-2

Writing COAST Goals

Remember that you should de-emphasize the treatment media in both your observations and your goal statements. Rewrite the following goal statements to emphasize change in occupational performance that you want to see and to de-emphasize the treatment interventions.

1. *Client will make a clock independently using the appropriate materials by anticipated discharge in 1 week.*

2. *Consumer will stay in his chair without reminders and spend at least 30 minutes lacing the leather billfold during the 45-minute craft group session within 2 weeks.*

Worksheet 11-3

SOAPing Your Note

Indicate in which section of the SOAP note you would place each of these statements.

_____ *Client supine → sit in bed* $\bigcirc$I.

_____ *Client moved kitchen items from counter to cabinet* $\bigcirc$I *using* $\bigcirc$L *hand.*

_____ *Decreased coordination, strength, sensation, and proprioception in* $\bigcirc$L *hand create safety risks in home management tasks.*

_____ *Client reports that his fingers are stiff this morning and that he is having trouble handling small items like buttons.*

_____ *↑ of 15 minutes in activity tolerance for UE activities permits client to prepare a light meal* $\bigcirc$I.

_____ *Child participated in 60-minute eval. of hand function in OT clinic.*

_____ *Decreased proprioception and motor planning limit* $\bigcirc$I *in upper body dressing.*

_____ *Continue retrograde massage to* $\bigcirc$R *hand for edema control.*

_____ *Correct identification of inappropriate positioning 100% of time indicates memory WFL.*

_____ *Client reports that she cannot remember hip precautions.*

_____ *Veteran would benefit from further instruction to incorporate total hip precautions into lower body dressing, bathing, and toileting.*

_____ *Client's improvement with repetition indicates good potential for successful access of augmentative communication device using eye gaze.*

_____ *Client did not make eye contact during group session.*

_____ *Client wrote check for correct amount to pay electric bill with 2 verbal cues.*

_____ *Client's request to take breaks demonstrates awareness of her limitations in endurance.*

_____ *Client completed weight shifts of trunk X 10 in each of anterior, posterior, left, and right lateral directions in preparation for standing to perform IADLs.*

_____ *3+ muscle grade of* $\bigcirc$R *wrist extension this week shows good progress toward goals.*

_____ *Continue OT 3x/wk. for 2 weeks to address cognitive impairments that impact safe performance of IADLs.*

_____ *Unkempt appearance in mock interview situation indicates poor judgment and self-concept.*

WORKSHEET 11-4

Writing the "S"—Subjective

The subjective section of your note contains the client's perception of the situation.

Inexperienced therapists sometimes list anything important the client has said about his or her condition. In the example below, all of the information is relevant, but does not form a coherent whole. This is not wrong and is better than reporting irrelevant data, but it is less skillful than reporting an organized and coherent summary of what the client had to say. Most of this client's comments have to do with transfers.

S: *Client told OT she has really bad arthritis in her right shoulder and Ⓛ knee.*
    Client rates pain at the site of her Ⓡ BKA as 8 out of 10.
    Client said, "It hurts to stand on my left leg."
    Client stated, "It [sliding board] needs to be moved further up on the seat."
    When asked if she was OK after the transfer, she said, "I'm just tired."
    Client stated, "I'm through," and requested help to get closer to the bed.
    When client transferred to the bed for dressing tasks, she said, "This is the hardest part."
    Client stated she prefers to transfer toward the Ⓡ side so she can push off with her Ⓛ LE and avoid bumping her Ⓡ BKA on the tire-rim of the w/c.

Write a more concise version of this "S," remembering to leave yourself out:

S:

WORKSHEET 11-5

"O"—Writing Good Opening Lines

Rewrite the following opening sentences to show how your skill as an OT is important in each situation.

1. *Client seen in room for 45 minutes for self-care activities.*

   Additional information: Client is on total hip precautions, which raises safety concerns during mobility, especially during toilet transfer. Adaptive equipment is available if needed.

2. *Client seen at workshop for 1 hr. to work on job skills.*

   Additional information: Client has deficits in sequencing tasks, which ↓ his ability to work Ⓘ. Ⓑ coordination problems interfere with client completing essential job function of opening/closing boxes. Sensory registration deficits contribute to client's high distractibility during task completion.

3. *Client seen bedside for 30 minutes for morning dressing.*

   Additional information: Deficits include ↓ balance and ↓ Ⓑ motor control of UEs that ↓ ability to safely complete ADL activities and use a manual w/c for mobility during ADLs.

4. *Client seen in kitchen for 1 hr. to work on Ⓘ in cooking.*

   Additional information: Client's problems include decreased dynamic standing balance and inattention of affected UE, which raise safety concerns.

WORKSHEET 11-6

"O"—Being Specific About Assist Levels

Do each of the following statements include the **specific part of the task** requiring assistance?

____ *Client required max Ⓐ x 2 bed → bedside commode and bed → w/c; Ⓓ for pericare.*

____ *Child required HOH Ⓐ to stay in the lines when following path with crayon.*

____ *Client needed mod verbal cues to participate in discussion during life skills group.*

____ *Resident needed min Ⓐ to don sock due to pain.*

WORKSHEET 11-7

Revising the "O"

Rather than rewriting this note to improve it, just write down your suggestions for what it needs to make it better.

O: **Toilet transfers**: *max Ⓐ*
  Toileting: *max Ⓐ 2° inability to support self c̄ Ⓛ arm and to dress*
  UE dressing: *min Ⓐ, verbal cues, set-up, Ⓘ in pulling shirt over head*
  LE dressing: *min Ⓐ pants to hips; max Ⓐ pants to waist*
    modified Ⓘ to don Ⓛ shoe (elastic laces); modified Ⓘ to don Ⓡ shoe
  Ⓡ hand status:
    Ⓡ fingers: small spasticity (index finger greatest amount)
    Thumb: CMC joint painful in abd & flex.
    Ⓡ wrist: flaccid

✦

✦

✦

✦

WORKSHEET 11-8

Differentiating Between Observations and Assessments

Identify which of these statements are **observations** and which are **assessments**. Remember that an observation tells you what the client did. An assessment will tell you how the contributing factor that is a problem impacts an area of occupation.

_____ *Client is unable to don AFO and shoe Ⓘ for ambulation.*

_____ *Inability to don AFO and shoe Ⓘ prevent client from ambulating safely around the house for IADL performance in order to live alone.*

_____ *Decreased sensory tolerance limits the client's attention to task in the classroom.*

_____ *Client required verbal cues to stay on task due to decreased sensory tolerance.*

_____ *Client was unable to incorporate breathing and energy conservation techniques, requiring several prompts to complete task.*

_____ *Inability to incorporate breathing techniques and energy conservation techniques into basic ADL tasks s̄ verbal prompts limits her ability to live alone Ⓘ p̄ discharge.*

The following statements are **observations** of something the OT saw the client do. Reword them so that they become **assessments**.

1. *Client demonstrated difficulty with laundry and cooking tasks due to memory and sequencing deficits.*

2. *Client unable to complete homemaking tasks or basic self-care activities independently due to decreased endurance and not following hip precautions.*

3. *After the use of behavioral modification techniques, client displayed courteous behavior for the remainder of the treatment session.*

WORKSHEET 11-9

Problems, Progress, and Rehab Potential

Mr. Y is a 68-year-old male who had a Ⓛ CVA 1 week ago. His Ⓡ UE is getting some return, and OT was ordered yesterday. Your colleague who assessed Mr. Y yesterday is out sick today, and you are beginning treatment with him. Her initial note stated that his activity tolerance was less than 1 minute and she was not sure how much aphasia was present.

O: *Client participated in 30-minute session in OT clinic to work on functional movements of Ⓡ UE, dynamic sitting balance, and cognitive skills. Client needed mod Ⓐ in shifting weight to get to edge of w/c and max verbal cues to use correct posture and shift feet during stand pivot transfer w/c → mat. Client required max verbal cues to initiate grasp of small beanbag. Client needed mod Ⓐ in reaching with Ⓡ UE. Client able to complete Ⓡ UE shoulder flexion required to toss beanbag ~2 ft with max verbal cues. Client demonstrated cognitive understanding of activity with mod verbal cues by stating desired goal to be achieved by accurate aim.*

Now assess the meaning of these data. Note the problems, progress, and rehab potential that you see for this client.

Problems:

Progress/Rehab Potential:

Now write an "A" that assesses how engagement in occupation is impacted. Include what the client would benefit from. Then write a "P" that describes your plan for this client.

A:

P:

WORKSHEET 11-10

Writing the "A" and "P"—The School Note

Now you will assess and plan for a school-age child. Remember that treatment in public school always relates to the child's educational performance. Cody is a second grader who is receiving OT in the public schools. He has several problems, including low muscle tone, which contributes to his upper body weakness and decreased proximal stability. At the time of the last note, he was able to achieve 70% accuracy in letter formation with verbal cues.

S: *Child stated, "This is hard!" during a bilateral coordination exercise requiring UE strength and stability.*

O: *Child participated in 30-minute session in school therapy room to improve oculomotor movements, fine motor skills required for handwriting, and upper body strength and stability necessary for dynamic UE function in the classroom.*

   Visual tracking*: Child visually tracked a moving object 4 times ⓡ → Ⓛ @ 40% accuracy and Ⓛ → ⓡ @ 20% accuracy. Child demonstrated 20% accuracy of eye convergence 4x staring 12" from nose and breaking at ~6" from nose.*

   UE coordination*: Child performed Ⓑ UE coordination activity (Zoom ball) at 80% accuracy with hyperextended knees and trunk movement to compensate for upper body weakness.*

   Handwriting*: Child able to write letters P, E, F, D, M, N, R from memory with 90% accuracy and 75% accuracy for staying in line boundaries with min verbal cues.*

What problems, progress, and/or rehab potential do you see for Cody?

Write your assessment and plan below.

A:

P:

WORKSHEET 11-11

Writing the "A" and "P"—Mr. S's Communication Skills

Mr. S is a 35-year-old male who is in a maximum security unit in a state psychiatric facility. He has criminal charges against him for a violent crime but was sent to the state mental institution rather than to prison. His current diagnosis is schizophrenia, r/o personality disorder. Today he participated in assertion group.

S: *Mr. S stated he knows what assertion is, but reports, "manipulation and aggression have always worked better for me." When asked to explain assertion, Mr. S stated, "The problem with that is the sugar and fruit in the cake."*

O: *Mr. S attended 1-hr. assertion group this date for skilled instruction and role play activities to improve assertion and effective self-expression skills. Mr. S was on time to the group, neatly dressed with hair combed. He was unable to correctly define assertion and did not respond to any of the three role-play activities, either by taking a role or by offering suggestions to others. During the role-play, Mr. S placed his head down and closed his eyes. Following the session, Mr. S quickly left the room.*

What problems, progress, and/or rehab potential do you see for Mr. S?

Write your assessment and plan below.

A:

P:

WORKSHEET 11-12

Revising the "Almost" Note

This note is **almost** good enough. In fact, it is quite good on the surface, but has major flaws in organization and clinical reasoning. Mrs. B is a 78-year-old female who has had a Ⓛ CVA and has Ⓡ hemiparesis. You do not have to rewrite this note, but as you read through it, keep track of suggestions that you have for improving it:

S: *Client reports stiffness in her Ⓡ hip, but improvement from previous pain. She states a preference for transferring to her left side. Client states she is willing to do "whatever it takes to get out of the hospital."*

O: *Client participated in 45-minute session in room to work on dressing and functional mobility during ADLs.*
__Transfer:__ Stand pivot transfer bed → w/c to left side SBA. Min Ⓐ with transfers w/c → toilet using grab bar.
__Mobility:__ Client rolled supine to Ⓡ side SBA with VCs to flex trunk. Client supine → sit SBA; sit → stand min Ⓐ; Ⓘ with w/c mobility.
__Dressing:__ Client donned shirt Ⓘ.
Client donned bra min Ⓐ with VCs while standing.
Client donned socks and shoes Ⓘ.
Client donned underwear and pants with min Ⓐ and VCs to stand with walker.
Client needs set-up for dressing activities.
__UE ROM:__ Ⓛ UE: WFL; Ⓡ UE: ↓ range in proximal shoulder flexion.
__Static standing:__ Client used walker for Ⓑ UE support with CGA.
__Dynamic standing:__ SBA with walker for balance

A: *Deficits noted in Ⓡ UE coordination, Ⓑ UE strength, and dynamic standing balance. Client Ⓘ in dressing EOB, but is min Ⓐ in dressing when standing with a walker. Ⓛ UE AROM is WFL but Ⓡ UE has deficits noted in shoulder flexion. Client needs SBA in bed mobility when rolling to unaffected side and min Ⓐ in sit → stand 2° ↓ UE strength. Client needs SBA for transfer to unaffected side in pivot transfer bed → w/c and min Ⓐ w/c → toilet. Client would benefit from skilled OT to continue UE strengthening and coordination exercise and to ↑ dynamic standing balance using walker in order to ↑ Ⓘ in ADLs.*

P: *Client to be seen 30 minutes b.i.d. for 2 weeks to continue work on dynamic standing balance during ADLs.*

What suggestions do you have for improving this note?

Chapter

Intervention Planning

Now that you know the basics of writing a SOAP note, we will back up a little and give some attention to the intervention planning on which your notes are based. You may recall from Chapter 1 that the *Framework-II* (AOTA, 2008b) describes both the domain and the process of occupational therapy. The first part of the occupational therapy process involves a thorough evaluation, including development of an occupational profile as well as analysis of occupational performance. Through the evaluation process, problems are identified, client priorities are determined, and targeted outcomes are developed.

The next step in the occupational therapy process is documenting the intervention plan, "a plan that will guide actions taken and that is developed in collaboration with the client. It is based on selected theories, frames of reference, and evidence" (AOTA, 2008b, p. 646). A frame of reference guides practice by delineating evaluation and intervention strategies for a specific area of practice (Crepeau et al., 2009b). The intervention strategies selected and the terminology used to describe those interventions will vary depending on the frames of reference used for a particular setting or client.

The *Framework-II* explains that interventions may be developed for a person, an organization, or a population. For purposes of learning, this manual will focus only on interventions targeted at individuals. However, the techniques described in this manual can be adapted for OTs who serve organizations and populations.

As explained in Chapter 10, the intervention plan is part of the "P" section of an evaluation SOAP note. We will discuss additional requirements related to evaluation documentation in Chapter 13. In this chapter, we will focus specifically on the goals, objectives, and intervention strategies contained in the intervention plan.

THE INTERVENTION PLANNING PROCESS

From the moment a referral is received, intervention planning begins in the mind of the therapist. A name, age, and reason for referral should stimulate an occupational therapist to begin reviewing in his or her mind the areas of occupation likely to be assessed, the areas of deficit that might be found, and the possible interventions that will benefit the client. Each individual is different of course, and there will be many variations, as well as some surprises as the assessment begins. The mental preparation for "*Clyde C, age 68, Ⓛ CVA, evaluate and treat*" takes a therapist on a mental journey along one road of thought, whereas "*Brooke J, age 4, ADHD, evaluate and treat*" takes the therapist mentally down a different pathway. From day one, a good therapist also begins discharge planning based on the client's occupational profile, prior level of performance, and probable discharge placement.

The *Guidelines for Documentation of Occupational Therapy* (AOTA, 2008a, p. 686) identify the components that should be included in an intervention plan:
- Client name and demographic information
- Measurable, occupation-based goals and objectives
- Intervention approaches and types of interventions to be used

Gateley CA, Borcherding S. *Documentation Manual for Occupational Therapy: Writing SOAP Notes, 3rd Edition* (pp. 143-156)
© 2012 SLACK Incorporated

✦ Service delivery mechanisms including provider, location, and frequency/duration

✦ Plan for discharge

✦ Outcome measures

✦ Professionals responsible for plan and date of plan development, review, or modification

The initial evaluation and intervention plan is written in whatever format the facility uses, and this will vary depending on practice setting. In earlier chapters, you learned how to write functional problem statements and how to address those problems by writing long-term and short-term goals, or objectives. Now we will discuss how to select intervention approaches and specific strategies to address the identified problems and to assist the client in meeting the established goals.

The *Framework-II* (AOTA, 2008b) outlines the various intervention approaches that may be used in occupational therapy:

✦ Health promotion to enrich activities and enhance performance

✦ Establishment of skills not yet developed or remediation/restoration of impaired skills

✦ Maintenance of performance capabilities, assuming that performance would decrease without intervention (Note: The word *maintain* is a red-flag word for reviewers; when documenting this approach, it is essential to elaborate on how the lack of OT services would lead to a significant decrease in occupational performance for the client. Examples include interventions for individuals with progressive disorders, such as Parkinson's Disease or macular degeneration, that help the individuals continue to function as independently as possible in the least restrictive environment.)

✦ Modification of context or activity through compensatory techniques or adaptation

✦ Prevention of occupational performance problems for clients with or without a disability

The intervention approaches listed above are closely tied to the client's targeted outcomes. These approaches describe **what** you hope to accomplish through occupational therapy intervention.

The *Framework-II* also lists the specific types of occupational therapy interventions that may be implemented:

✦ Therapeutic use of self

✦ Therapeutic use of occupations and activities
  • Preparatory methods
  • Purposeful activity
  • Occupation-based intervention

✦ Consultation process

✦ Education process

✦ Advocacy

The types of OT interventions described above explain **how** you will help the client meet the targeted outcomes. Let's take a closer look at each of these interventions.

THERAPEUTIC USE OF SELF

Therapeutic use of self is "an occupational therapy practitioner's planned use of his or her personality, insights, perceptions, and judgments as part of the therapeutic process" (AOTA, 2008b, p. 653). While often not specified in an intervention plan, therapeutic use of self is inherent in any OT session and is one of the hallmarks of our profession.

THERAPEUTIC USE OF OCCUPATIONS AND ACTIVITIES

This type of intervention involves selecting specific activities to meet the client's goals while taking into consideration client factors, activity demands, and context. This includes the use of adaptive devices and environmental modifications. There are three different levels of therapeutic use of occupations and activities:

1. *Preparatory methods*: Methods used to prepare the client for occupational performance. Examples include physical agent modalities, use of splints, strengthening exercises, and sensory stimulation.

2. *Purposeful activity*: Activities that focus on the development of specific skills to enhance engagement in occupation. Examples include learning the use of adaptive equipment for dressing, learning tub transfers, and participating in role play to develop social skills.

3. *Occupation-based intervention*: Client-directed occupations that match the client's goals. Examples include completing morning ADLs, taking the city bus to the grocery store, playing on the school playground, and applying for a job.

One error that students and new therapists sometimes make is getting stuck on the preparatory methods and failing to move toward purposeful activity and occupation-based intervention. If you keep in mind your client's occupation-based goals, you should be able to develop a comprehensive intervention plan that includes all three types of intervention described above.

CONSULTATION PROCESS

Consultation involves the practitioner using his or her knowledge and expertise to collaborate with the client and/or others involved in the daily activities of the client. Using this type of intervention, the OT makes recommendations for identified problems but does not directly carry out the interventions. Examples include consulting with a manufacturing plant to design more ergonomic work stations or consulting with a classroom teacher to reduce the visual and auditory distractions for a child who is overly sensitive to such input.

EDUCATION PROCESS

This "involves imparting knowledge and information about occupation, health, and participation and does not result in the actual performance of the occupation/activity" (AOTA, 2008b, p. 654). Examples include educating a client about available community services after discharge or instructing nursing staff about positioning and transfer techniques for clients with hemiplegia.

ADVOCACY

Advocacy involves collaborating with individuals, organizations, and populations to promote occupational justice and help them obtain the resources needed for occupational participation. Examples include helping to justify to an insurance company the medical necessity of a child's power wheelchair or serving on a committee that encourages application of universal design principles in new city buildings.

OTHER CONSIDERATIONS

In addition to being aware of the different intervention approaches and techniques, there are other factors that must be considered when setting goals and selecting interventions to meet those goals.

ESTIMATING REHAB POTENTIAL

Rehab potential should always be stated as good or excellent for the goals you want the client to accomplish. If your client's rehab potential is not good or excellent for the stated goals, you may need to select smaller, more incremental goals. There is not much point in setting and working toward goals that the client does not have a good chance of accomplishing. Estimating rehab potential as *poor*, *fair*, or *guarded* is a red flag to reviewers, and they may be reluctant to set aside health care dollars for someone who is unlikely to benefit from your intervention.

> Note: "Rehab potential" does **not** mean independence. It means potential to reach the goals you have set or potential for the client to make significant change.

SELECTING MEANINGFUL INTERVENTION STRATEGIES

Since selecting strategies and treatment media is a daily task for an occupational therapist, it can seem to an inexperienced therapist almost like reinventing the wheel to select different strategies for each individual client. One of the striking differences between OT and other disciplines is the way in which strategies and media are selected to meet the client's goals. In OT, the selected activities must be meaningful to the individual client (Crepeau et al., 2009a). OT is a process of creative problem solving with each client in each area of occupation. What is meaningful to one client may not be meaningful to another.

Even the most basic task such as dressing may not seem meaningful to some clients. A person with tetraplegia who has a personal attendant, for example, may never need to dress himself and may consider it an enormous waste of time to be required to learn to do so. However, he may be very motivated to learn how to use a power wheelchair operated with head controls in order to be independent with mobility needed to re-engage in social participation with his friends. Some clients will never need to balance a checkbook, while others may not be able to return to living independently without this skill. The difference between competent and exceptional OT may well lie in the ability to find meaningful activities and design these into intervention strategies.

The OT asks questions like these:

+ What do you want to be able to do?
+ What keeps you from being able to do that?
+ What are the possible options for making that happen?

The options for intervention strategies may include teaching new skills or patterns, working to increase client factors (ROM, strength, endurance), or modifying the environment (context) to improve occupational performance. OTs consider doing things in many different ways. The creativity of the individual therapist blossoms in intervention planning. How many ways are there to get light into a room if the client can no longer manage a light switch? How many activities that require wrist extension could be adapted to work toward a long-term goal of returning to an assembly line position that requires increased AROM of the wrist? Would any of these activities qualify as meaningful to this client?

The treatment media used in occupational therapy is also different from that used by other disciplines. OTs often use common household objects to accomplish tasks or activities related to occupational performance. For example, the client's own clothing is a common treatment media. The clothes may be used for dressing to teach the client to don clothing; for folding to have the client do a meaningful activity while increasing standing tolerance; or for hanging in a closet to help the client increase AROM at the shoulder. The approach would depend on what the client will need to do in the setting to which he or she will be discharged. An experienced occupational therapist can find many different uses for common household objects. The same mesh sponge that is used to wash dishes may be used for squeezing to develop grip strength or for throwing to develop AROM in the upper extremities.

Determining Frequency and Duration of Treatment

In Chapter 10, you learned that the frequency and duration of OT services vary greatly between settings and funding sources. It may seem impossible to a new therapist to estimate how much time will be needed to accomplish goals. With a little experience, you will find that you really can do it. Please remember that the intervention plan is made to be changed. If your original estimate does not turn out to be accurate, you change it as you find out how quickly your client progresses.

Clinical Pathways

A clinical pathway, also known as a *critical care pathway*, is "…a coordinated, multidisciplinary approach emphasizing the patient's functional recovery and restoration of quality of life…" (Koval & Cooley, 2005, p. 1058). The purpose of clinical pathways is to provide care in a cost-effective manner, essentially reducing the length of inpatient hospitalization. The clinical pathway includes a standardized intervention plan based on a predictable course of recovery.

In addition to standardizing intervention strategies and establishing check points along a time line, the use of a standard intervention plan is also more efficient by avoiding unnecessary time rewriting basically the same plan for routine treatment approaches. The standardized plan does allow for adaptations to accommodate individual client differences such as multiple diagnoses (e.g., knee replacement and multiple sclerosis).

Some diagnoses such as stroke are too complex to use a clinical pathway, while others are very compatible with a standardized approach to treatment. Clinical pathways are used most often following orthopedic surgeries including hip and knee replacements and various spinal procedures (laminectomies, discectomies, fusions, etc.). See Table 12-1 for an example of a clinical pathway.

Table 12-1

Clinical Pathway—Total Hip Replacement

POSTOPERATIVE DAY 1

- Initial OT evaluation, including transfer bed ↔ w/c
- Skilled instruction of hip precautions; provide handout
- Have pt. verbalize and demonstrate precautions during ADLs, within activity tolerance

POSTOPERATIVE DAY 2*

- Continue skilled instruction of hip precautions
- Assess adaptive equipment needs for dressing, toileting, bathing
- Procure necessary equipment via hospital procedures
- Practice lower body dressing, bedside commode transfer, grooming at sink in stance
- Begin UE strengthening if needed; introduce home program and have client demonstrate

POSTOPERATIVE DAY 3*

- Bathing assessment in tub or shower
- Practice transfer to toilet with riser or commode frame
- Practice car transfer in car simulator
- Provide home safety education (especially kitchen task if will be home alone) and have pt. practice as needed
- Reassess client's understanding of UE home exercise program

* Pt. may be discharged postoperative day 2, 3, or 4 depending on progress. If discharge is planned for postoperative day 2, all interventions listed for postoperative day 3 should also be covered on postoperative day 2. SNF referral may be made for those patients requiring a longer recovery period.

SAMPLE INTERVENTION PLAN

Client Name: Marge B   **DOB**: 3/24/1932   **Age**: 79
1° Dx: Ⓛ CVA   **2° Dx**: DM
Referring Physician: Dr. D   **Primary OT**: Charlet Q, OTR/L

Frequency/Duration: 30 minutes 2x/day for 3 weeks

Occupational Profile: Ms. B is a widow who lives with her daughter and grandson in a one-story house in a small town. Ms. B was Ⓘ in all ADL and IADL tasks before her CVA. She has never worked outside her home. She raised 7 children in the town where she now resides and takes pride in her ability to do homemaking tasks such as cooking, sewing, and decorating. She drives in her own small town, but is not comfortable driving long distances. She intends to return to the home she shares with her daughter and grandson and hopes to return to her PLOF.

Problem: Client requires mod Ⓐ in self-care due to inability to spontaneously use Ⓡ UE 2° Ⓛ CVA.

Long-Term Goal: Client will complete all ADL and IADL activities with modified Ⓘ within 3 weeks.

STG (Objective)	Interventions
STG #1: Client will complete grooming tasks using ® UE spontaneously as a functional assist within 1 week.	1. *Normalize tone through use of NDT approaches.* 2. *Instruct in sensory stimulation to affected side to ↓ neglect.* 3. *Weight bear on ® UE while engaged in functional activities that require weight shifts: sorting laundry, playing a board game, turning pages of a magazine.* 4. *Facilitate grasp and release for use of prehension; facilitate reach patterns through handling, joint approximation, guided resistance, and muscle stretch.* 5. *Provide activities that require ® UE as an assist (stabilizing tablet while writing, stabilizing toothpaste while removing lid, applying body lotion).*
STG #2: Client will dress self with min Ⓐ within 2 weeks using ® UE as a functional assist.	1. *Instruct in adaptive dressing techniques.* 2. *Instruct in use of ® UE to stabilize shirt while buttoning, assist in pulling up pants, holding onto bra while hooking in front.* 3. *Instruct in adaptive equipment as needed: long shoe horn, elastic shoelaces, reacher, or dressing stick.* 4. *Facilitate trunk control and balance in weight shifts forward and backward, side to side, and in rotational patterns in preparation for and throughout dressing activity as needed.*
STG #3: Client will complete light meal preparation and clean-up with SBA for safety within 3 weeks.	1. *In collaboration with client and family, adapt kitchen for safe accessibility and mobility.* 2. *Plan meal with attention to money management, organization, and sequencing of component tasks.* 3. *Instruct in functional mobility in kitchen to transport items while preparing lunch using gait patterns learned in PT. Use wheeled cart as needed for safe and efficient transport of items.* 4. *Instruct in correct and safe body mechanics in reaching items in refrigerator, on stove top, in oven, or in microwave, and in performing, sink, countertop, and cooking activities.* 5. *Instruct in energy conservation during meal preparation and clean-up.* 6. *Select and instruct in use of appropriate adaptive equipment for one-handedness as needed to peel and chop vegetables, open cans and jars.*

Note that the interventions planned for Ms. B include a combination of preparatory methods, purposeful activities, and occupation-based interventions.

COMMON ERRORS IN WRITING INTERVENTION PLANS

PROBLEM IDENTIFICATION

✦ Problems identified in the assessment are not addressed in the plan.
✦ Problems are not stated in terms of behavioral manifestations, areas of occupation, and contributing factors.
✦ The number of visits requested does not match the severity of the documented problems.

GOALS

+ Goals are not functional or do not focus on the reason for referral to occupational therapy.
+ Intervention plan does not focus on specific rehabilitation goals that will increase a client's ability to engage in meaningful occupation in the probable discharge environment.
+ Goals focus on the client participating in or cooperating with treatment (unless the client is in the habit of refusing treatment; more acceptable in mental health and behavioral health settings).
+ Goals are not measurable or do not have a target date for completion.

INTERVENTION STRATEGIES

+ Interventions do not focus on increasing functional behaviors in order to return the client to the least restrictive environment.
+ Interventions do not take into account the age, gender, and interests of the client or are not meaningful to the client.
+ Acquired skills are not transferred into more functional contexts in the client's life.
+ Intervention strategies focus too heavily on preparatory methods without progression toward purposeful activities and occupation-based interventions.

CLIENT INVOLVEMENT

+ The client is not involved in the treatment planning process. (Note: The client's signature on the intervention plan indicating that client has read it is not enough to indicate significant client involvement.)
+ Intervention plan does not reflect the client's strengths, desires, and preferences.

"CANNED" PLANS

+ "Canned" intervention plans reflect the same goals, objectives, and interventions for each client based on the diagnosis and services available rather than on client need. (Even clinical pathways need to be individualized to fit the client.)

WORKSHEET 12-1

Choosing Intervention Strategies

Intervention strategies do not stand alone. Strategies must be based on problems and long-term goals, and they must be purposeful to the client to be useful. However, for purposes of learning to generate possible strategies, we will suspend that requirement and think of as many ways as possible to meet a treatment objective. Consider the following example:

STG	Interventions
Client will complete basic ADL tasks with SBA while standing for 5-minute increments and taking rest breaks as needed by discharge date of 9/10/11.	1. *Set-up task to make coffee while standing at counter in the ADL kitchen.* 2. *Have client stand at the bathroom sink to complete face washing and tooth brushing.* 3. *Have client stand at a table to play a card game.* 4. *Instruct client to stand to retrieve clothing from closet when dressing in the AM.* 5. *Have client stand to look out window to watch birds eat the food she has put out.* 6. *Instruct client to stand while watering plants in windowsill of dining room.*

Using the STG below, think of as many intervention strategies as possible that would help the client meet this goal.

STG	Interventions
Client will be ① in managing financial affairs within 3 weeks.	

WORKSHEET 12-2

Writing the Assessment and Intervention Plan: The Case of Georgia S

Name: *Georgia S*   **Age**: *87*   **Sex**: *F*   **Physician**: *L. Yang, MD*
Dx: Ⓛ *SDH on 6/1/11; hx. of HTN, hearing loss*
Onset: *6/1/11*   **Date of Referral**: *6/11/11*   **Date of Eval**: *6/12/11*

Background data and beginning occupational profile: *Prior to her stroke, Georgia had been living for the past 10 years with her unmarried daughter, Janice, who is 60 years old and works full-time. They live in a two-story house with the only bathroom on the second floor. Georgia was in acute care and has just been transferred to a rehabilitation center. She expresses a desire to return to her daughter's home. Her daughter has concerns about being able to care for her mother at home. Georgia has Medicare as her only insurance coverage.*

S: *Client expressed frustration when having difficulty brushing teeth. Client c/o back pain 2/10 when standing for grooming. Client's daughter said that client was* Ⓘ *in self-care prior to her stroke but has not cooked or done housework for years; also stated that client has a hearing loss but no hearing aids.*

O: *Client participated in 45-minute OT session in room for initial evaluation.*
    Dressing/Grooming: *Client stood with CGA for 5 min while brushing teeth after set-up and 2 verbal cues. Client modified* Ⓘ *in donning/doffing socks with extra time. Client attempted to don* Ⓡ *sock using same technique for several minutes before being successful. Client did not attempt an alternative technique. Client donned/doffed gown with mod* Ⓐ *pulling the robe around her back and threading the* Ⓡ *UE into the sleeve. Client required four 30-second rest breaks during dressing activity due to fatigue.*
    Functional Mobility: *Client sit → stand SBA; mod* Ⓐ *needed for standing balance while managing clothing during bedside commode transfer. Client walked 3 ft. w/c → sink using walker with CGA.*
    UE ROM & Strength: *All UE AROM WNL except* Ⓑ *shoulder abduction and flexion which were WFL.* Ⓑ *UE strength 5/5 overall except 3/5 in* Ⓑ *shoulder flex. & abd.*
    Grip Strength: Ⓛ *37#,* Ⓡ *29#*
    Lateral Pinch: Ⓛ *9#;* Ⓡ *7.5#*   ***Tripod Pinch***: Ⓛ *7#;* Ⓡ *4#*
    Sensation: *Light touch and sharp/dull discrimination intact* Ⓑ. *Client correctly identified 1 of 4 objects in* Ⓡ *stereognosis test.*
    Coordination (9 Hole Peg Test): *Placing pegs* Ⓛ *37 secs,* Ⓡ *52 secs*
                        Removal Ⓛ *14 secs,* Ⓡ *26 secs*

Write the "A" and "P" as you learned in Chapters 9 and 10. Turn your problems into correctly worded problem statements. Identify the rehab potential you see for Ms. S. On the intervention plan, you will include some of these items as "strengths."

A:

P:

Strengths:

WORKSHEET 12-2 (CONTINUED)

Writing the Assessment and Intervention Plan: The Case of Georgia S

Functional Problem Statement #1:

Long-Term Goal #1:

STGs (Objectives)	Interventions
STG #1:	
STG #2:	

Functional Problem Statement #2:

Long-Term Goal #2:

STGs (Objectives)	Interventions
STG #1:	
STG #2:	

Discharge Plan:

Signature:

WORKSHEET 12-3

Planning Interventions Using Groups—Heather's Suicide Attempt

In some practice settings, clients are seen primarily in groups rather than individually. This strategy has the advantage of using peer feedback and support as part of the treatment process. It also provides challenges for the therapist in finding ways to structure the group to meet the needs of all of the clients attending. Below is a description of a client who is being seen in a psychiatric unit where intervention strategies generally take place in groups. After you read about this client, choose intervention strategies to use for her in each of the groups she attends.

Heather S is a 40-year-old, unemployed woman with a psychiatric disability who recently separated from her husband. She has two children, a daughter age 22 and a son age 18. Heather was admitted through the emergency department post ingestion of an overdose of psychiatric medications. She was lavaged and admitted briefly to a medical unit, where she was stabilized in 8 hours and transferred to the psychiatric unit with a diagnosis of depression.

Heather was sexually abused from the ages of 10 to 13 by an uncle who lived in the home where she was one of five children. Her estranged husband abuses alcohol and is emotionally abusive to Heather when he has been drinking. Heather married him when she was 18 years old and pregnant with her first child. They have been married 21 years.

Heather reports that she has trouble with expression of anger. She doesn't always know she is getting angry, and then "explodes" in ways that are destructive to herself, others, and property. She also says she is having a lot of trouble making decisions, and that her husband has traditionally made decisions for her. She says that she "just can't think" and has difficulty paying attention to anything for more than a few minutes. For example, she is unable to complete a magazine article she is reading. Her appearance is disheveled, her hair is uncombed, and she is wearing no makeup or jewelry. She picks at her clothing while she talks to you, looking at the floor and making little eye contact.

The problem areas identified by the treatment team include anger, decision making, and poor self-esteem with suicidal ideas. Heather's anticipated length of stay is 4 days. The psychiatric unit provides an array of individual and group treatment sessions. In addition to the medication group and the individual sessions done by the psychiatrist, there is group therapy provided by the social worker, and an evening wrap-up group provided by nursing. OT provides 3 groups per day:

✦ Goals group ½ hour each morning

✦ Stress management group 1 hour daily

✦ IADL group 1 hour daily

The IADL group covers topics such as money management, parenting, assertion skills, and other IADL skills depending on the needs and issues that are common to the current clients. For example, if several clients have difficulty expressing anger in useful ways, you could use IADL group time to address anger management.

In a psychiatric unit, the treatment plan is usually multidisciplinary. Because we are working with a 4-day length of stay and a multidisciplinary treatment plan, we will not write objectives for each of Heather's goals. Heather will be seen in OT groups every day while she is in the hospital. In this worksheet, you will decide how to use the group time to Heather's best advantage in meeting her established goals. Keep in mind that your interventions will include not only the activities you plan to use, but also your **therapeutic use of self** with Heather—the ways you might plan to interact with her and the behaviors you want to model.

WORKSHEET 12-3 (CONTINUED)

Planning Interventions Using Groups—Heather's Suicide Attempt

Problem #1: Exacerbation of depressive symptoms resulting in a suicide attempt.

LTG #1: By anticipated discharge in 4 days, Heather will demonstrate improved self-esteem by verbally identifying strengths, caring for her appearance, making eye contact when interacting with others, and developing a plan for coping with suicidal thoughts.

Interventions	
Goals Group	
Stress Management Group	
IADL Group	

Problem #2: Stress related to recent role changes results in Heather's inability to concentrate and make decisions for her daily life.

LTG #2: Heather will apply a decision-making strategy to her two most important current life decisions by discharge in 4 days.

Interventions	
Goals Group	
Stress Management Group	
IADL Group	

Problem #3: Inability to manage anger constructively resulting in behaviors that damage self, relationships, and property.

LTG #3: By anticipated discharge in 4 days, Heather independently will identify potential anger triggers, her physical reactions to being angry, and develop a plan to prevent escalation and destructive behaviors.

Interventions	
Goals Group	
Stress Management Group	
IADL Group	

13

Documenting Different Stages of Service Delivery

Different stages of the occupational therapy process require you to write different types of notes. The setting and a client's funding source may also impact the type of note required. As discussed in Chapter 1, the occupational therapy process of service delivery consists of evaluation, intervention, and outcomes. The *Guidelines for Documentation of Occupational Therapy* (AOTA, 2008a, p. 684) outlines the reports for each part of the service delivery process:

+ Evaluation
  + Evaluation or screening report
  + Re-evaluation report
+ Intervention
  + Intervention plan
  + OT service contacts
  + Progress report
  + Transition plan
+ Outcomes
  + Discharge/discontinuation report

In this chapter, we will review the specific content required for each type of note and provide examples for your reference. Please be aware that the information presented in this chapter is a summary of information found in the *Guidelines for Documentation of Occupational Therapy* (AOTA, 2008a). This document, like all AOTA *Official Documents*, is updated approximately every 5 years. To be certain you are following current standards, you should refer to the most recent document published in the *American Journal of Occupational Therapy*. The document is also available at www.aota.org for AOTA members.

FUNDAMENTAL ELEMENTS OF ALL DOCUMENTATION

The *Guidelines for Documentation of Occupational Therapy* lists several elements that are essential to all types of documentation:

+ Client's full name and case number (if applicable) on each page of documentation
+ Date and type of occupational therapy contact
+ Identification of type of documentation, agency, and department name
+ OT practitioner's signature with a minimum of first name or initial, last name, and professional designation
+ When applicable on notes or reports, signature of the recorder directly at the end of the note without space left between the body of the note and the signature

Gateley CA, Borcherding S. *Documentation Manual for Occupational Therapy: Writing SOAP Notes, 3rd Edition* (pp. 157-168)
© 2012 SLACK Incorporated

✦ Countersignature by an OT on documentation written by students and OTAs when required by law or the facility

✦ Acceptable terminology defined within the boundaries of the setting

✦ Abbreviations usage as acceptable within the boundaries of the setting

✦ When no facility requirements are listed, errors corrected by drawing a single line through an error and by initialing the correction (liquid correction fluid and erasures are not acceptable)

✦ Adherence to professional standards of technology, when used to document OT services

✦ Disposal of records within law or agency requirements

✦ Compliance with confidentiality standards

✦ Compliance with agency or legal requirements of storage of records

Reprinted with permission from *Guidelines for Documentation of Occupational Therapy* (AOTA, 2008a).

Note: In the next section, you will find a list of elements to be included in each type of OT note. While each **category** in the list must be present, the **specific elements** in each category will vary depending on facility requirements and your client's individual situation. These lists are intended to be a reference for you as you learn to write notes for different stages of treatment.

EVALUATION

EVALUATION OR SCREENING REPORT

After a referral for OT is received for a client, you begin gathering information about the client's occupational history as well as other factors that impact his or her engagement in occupation. This is the beginning of the occupational profile, which will tell you what the client needs and wants from OT. First you collect data from the client, the family, the chart, and any other pertinent sources. Then you select and administer any standardized tests or survey instruments that will help you determine more specifically what contributing factors support or hinder participation in occupations. You also use your clinical observation skills to analyze occupational performance. Finally, you compile all of your data into a comprehensive report. Suggested content with examples includes the following:

✦ *Client information*: Name/agency, date of birth, gender, health status, applicable medical/educational/developmental diagnoses, precautions, and contraindications

✦ *Referral information*: Date and source of referral, services requested, reason for referral, funding source, and anticipated length of service

✦ *Occupational profile*: Client's reason for seeking occupational therapy services, current areas of occupation that are successful and problematic, contexts and environments that support and hinder occupations, medical/educational/work history, occupational history (e.g., patterns of living, interest, values), client priorities, and targeted outcomes

✦ *Assessments used and results*: Types of assessments used and results (e.g., interviews, record reviews, observations, standardized or nonstandardized assessments), and confidence in test results

✦ *Analysis of occupational performance*: Description of and judgment about performance skills, performance patterns, contexts and environments, features of the activities, and client factors that facilitate and inhibit performance

✦ *Summary and analysis*: Interpretation and summary of data as it is related to occupational profile and referring concern

✦ *Recommendation*: Judgment regarding appropriateness of occupational therapy services or other services

Reprinted with permission from *Guidelines for Documentation of Occupational Therapy* (AOTA, 2008a).

In some cases, you may be asked to perform a screening rather than a thorough evaluation process. In such cases, you would document the limited areas of occupation and occupational performance that are applicable to the client and the situation.

Most facilities still using paper documentation provide a form for an initial evaluation report, and evaluation results are recorded on the form along with comments and observations. Some facilities use the same form for re-evaluation and discharge reports so that the evaluation material does not have to be rewritten. Figure 13-1 shows the evaluation and discharge report form from Capital Region Medical Center in Jefferson City, Missouri, so that you can see what might be included on a good facility form. Because this is an acute care facility, there is an emphasis on some areas of occupation (ADLs) over others (play or social participation).

Note also that this form includes the intervention plan. Although the intervention plan represents a different stage in the OT process (intervention), it is often included along with the initial evaluation report since a plan must be in place before treatment is continued. Therefore, we will present the guidelines for the intervention plan and the corresponding example in conjunction with the initial evaluation.

INTERVENTION PLAN

Chapter 12 provided a detailed discussion about the purpose and process of intervention planning, as well as several examples. The suggested content for an intervention plan includes the following:

- ✦ *Client information*: Name/agency, date of birth, gender, diagnosis, precautions, and contraindications
- ✦ *Intervention goals*: Measurable goals and short-term objectives directly related to the client's ability and need to engage in desired occupations
- ✦ *Intervention approaches and types of interventions to be used*: Intervention approaches that include create/promote, establish/restore, maintain, modify, and prevent; types of interventions that include consultation process, education process, advocacy, therapeutic use of occupations or activities, and therapeutic use of self
- ✦ *Service delivery mechanisms*: Service provider, service location, and frequency and duration of services
- ✦ *Plan for discharge*: Discontinuation criteria, location of discharge, and follow-up care
- ✦ *Outcomes measures*: Outcomes that include improved occupational performance, adaptation, role competence, improved health and wellness, prevention of further difficulties, improved quality of life, self-advocacy, and occupational justice
- ✦ *Professionals responsible and date of plan*: Names and positions of persons overseeing plan, date plan was developed, and date when plan was modified or reviewed

Reprinted with permission from *Guidelines for Documentation of Occupational Therapy* (AOTA, 2008a).

Occupational Therapy Initial Evaluation Report

Name: Rosa S   *Age*: 68   *Gender*: F   *Physician*: Dr. Grantham
Date of Onset: 2/1/11   *Date of Admission*: 2/2/11   *Insurance*: Medicare & supplement
Referral Data: Client referred by Dr. Grantham on 2/2/11 for evaluation and treatment.
1° Dx: Ⓡ CVA r/o OBS   *2° Dx*: Diabetes   *Date of Eval*: 2/3/11   *Time*: 10:00 am

Occupational Profile: Client was admitted after a fall resulting in confusion and left-sided weakness. Prior to admission, she was living alone in a one-story home and was Ⓘ in all ADLs. Client is a retired librarian and states she values her independence and fully intends to return to her own home. Hobbies include mostly sedentary activities such as sewing, reading, and playing cards with friends. Daughter works during the day, lives two blocks away, and is willing to visit daily and assist with transportation, but cannot provide 24-hr supervision.

S: Client stated, "I'll work hard in rehab. I need to get home."

O: Client participated in 60-minute evaluation in room and shower room for Mini-Mental Status Examination (MMSE), and evaluation of ADLs, functional mobility, and contributing factors (MMT, AROM).
         Bathing: Upper body: min Ⓐ to sequence task. Lower body: min Ⓐ except max Ⓐ to reach perineal area and feet.
         Dressing: Seated in chair with arms, min Ⓐ to maintain dynamic balance when bending, mod Ⓐ to initiate donning bra, and max Ⓐ to reach feet. Verbal cues needed for sequencing and environmental orientation.
         Toileting: Min Ⓐ to obtain tissue and manage clothing, verbal cues to flush.
         Transfers: CGA with verbal cues for safety/proper arm placement sit to stand; min Ⓐ from low surfaces.
         Bed Mobility: Rolls & supine ↔ sit SBA for safety.
         Static Standing Balance: CGA
         Activity Tolerance: <10 min tolerance for any activity with physical/mental challenges.
         Motor Planning/Perception: WFL
         Cognition: Score of 17/20 on MMSE. Sequencing problems during dressing tasks noted. Client unable to fasten bra in back; required verbal cues to fasten in front.

CAPITAL REGION MEDICAL CENTER
OCCUPATIONAL THERAPY
☐ **INITIAL EVALUATION** ☐ **DISCHARGE SUMMARY**

DIAGNOSIS _____ ONSET: _____

MED. HX: _____

_____ CODE STATUS: _____

RELEVANT SURG. PROC.: _____

REFERRAL DATE: _____ DATE: _____

REFERRING PHYSICIAN: _____ MEDICARE #: _____

ACTIVITIES OF DAILY LIVING   REHAB POTENTIAL: _____

DRESSING Put on & remove the following	INDEP	SBA	MIN. ASSIST	MOD. ASSIST	MAX. ASSIST	ADAPT. EQUIP.	COMMENTS/ADAPTIVE EQUIPMENT ISSUED
front opening shirt							
pull on shirt							
underwear							
bra							
pants/slacks							
socks/hose							
shoes							
manage fasteners							
braces/splints/prosthesis							
GROOMING/HYGIENE							
sponge bath							
tub/shower bath							
shave							
comb hair							
brushing teeth							
opens jars/bottles							
make-up							
EATING							
drink from cup/glass							
feeds self							
cuts meat							

ROM — **UPPER EXTREMITY ROM & STRENGTH**

ACTIVE LEFT	PASSIVE LEFT	ACTIVE RIGHT	PASSIVE RIGHT			STRENGTH L	R
				SHOULDER:	Elevation		
					Flexion		
					Abduction		
					Horizontal Abduction		
					Horizontal Adduction		
					Internal Rotation		
					External Rotation		
				ELBOW:	Flexion		
					Extension		
					Supination		
					Pronation		
				WRIST:	Flexion		
				Shoulder Subluxation L	R		
				UE Edema L	R		
				Pain L	R		

PERTINENT FINDINGS

Wears glasses_____ Dentures_____ Hearing_____

MUSCLE TONE/UPPER EXTREMITIES

Hypotonic_____ Normal_____ Hypertonic_____
Comments_____

UPPER EXTREMITY SENSATION

SENSATION	Intact	Impaired	Absent
Light touch			
Sharp/Dull			
Temperature			
Proprioception			
Stereognosis			

COORDINATION/UPPER EXTREMITIES

Tremors_____ Apraxia_____ Ataxic_____
                              Impaired   WNL

	Impaired	WNL
Gross Motor		
Fine Motor		
9 Hole Peg Test	L	R
Grip Strength	L	R
Lateral Pinch	L	R
Tripod Pinch	L	R
Hand Dominance	L	R

SURVIVAL SKILLS	Indep.	Min. Assist	Mod. Assist	Max. Assist
Phone Book Usage				
Money Mngmt.				
Situational Problem Solving				
Homemaking				

ORIENTED TO:

Person_____ Place_____
Time: Month_____ Day_____ Year_____
Situation_____

COMMUNICATION/COGNITION

	YES	NO
Verbal		
Understandable		
Appropriate		
Perseveration		
Follows Simple Commands		
Reads		
Writes		

2,605,003 (9/99) INIT. EVAL/DISCHG. SUM. (FRONT)

PERCEPTION

A. R/L Neglect_____
                              Impaired   WNL
B. Body Schema
C. Discrimination
       Shape
       Size
       Color
D. Visual Perception

Overall Endurance   WFL_____
                              Fair_____
                              Poor_____

Figure 13-1. Evaluation and discharge report form. (Reprinted with permission of Capital Region Medical Center, Jefferson City, MO.) (continued)

HOME SITUATION: _____

LIVING ARRANGEMENTS: (PT ADDRESS) _____

HOME TYPE: _____

PRIOR FUNCTIONAL INDEP.: _____

_____

_____

LEISURE INTERESTS: _____

ADAPTIVE EQUIP.: _____

COMMENTS: _____

_____

_____

_____

PATIENT / FAMILY GOALS: _____

❏ INITIAL ASSESSMENT (PROBLEMS / STRENGTHS)   ❏ DISCHARGE STATUS OF SHORT / LONG TERM GOALS

_____

_____

_____

_____

_____

PLAN: _____

SHORT-TERM GOALS - ESTIMATED TIME TO ACHIEVE: _____

_____

_____

_____

_____

_____

❏ LONG-TERM GOALS - ESTIMATED TIME TO ACHIEVE: ❏ RECOMMENDATIONS:

_____

_____

_____

_____

_____

❏ Yes   ❏ No   **Patient has participated in evaluation process and agrees with treatment plan as stated above.**

Therapist _____   Date_____

I have reviewed and agree with the treatment plan as stated above.

Physician Signature _____   Date_____

2.605.003 (9/99) OT INITIAL EVALUATION/DISCHARGE SUMMARY (BACK)

Figure 13-1 (continued). Evaluation and discharge report form. (Reprinted with permission of Capital Region Medical Center, Jefferson City, MO.)

UE AROM: WFL for all Ⓑ UE movements, except ¾ range Ⓛ shoulder flex/abd against gravity.
MMT: Ⓡ UE 4+/5 throughout; Ⓛ UE 3+/5 throughout
Strength: Grip: Ⓡ 42 lbs, Ⓛ 21 lbs   Lateral Pinch: Ⓡ 14 lbs, Ⓛ 6 lbs
          Tripod Pinch: Ⓡ 12 lbs, Ⓛ 5 lbs   Tip Pinch: Ⓡ 8 lbs, Ⓛ 2 lbs
Sensation: Ⓡ UE intact; Ⓛ UE light touch, pain, temperature intact; stereognosis 3 of 5.

A: Client's poor problem-solving skills (needing cues to sequence activity and inability to initiate alternative way to don bra) and need for verbal cues to initiate some ADL tasks limit her ability to manage ADLs and IADLs Ⓘ. Decreased AROM and strength in Ⓛ UE along with slow response to cognitive tasks, decreased ability to sequence tasks, and decreased short-term memory raise safety concerns in returning to independent living. Client's motivation indicates good potential for returning to modified Ⓘ in ADL activities. Client would benefit from environmental cues to orient her to environment, facilitation of problem solving, sequencing activities, and activities to increase strength in Ⓛ UE.

P: Client will receive OT for 45-minute sessions 5x/wk for 2 wks to work toward increased independence with ADLs, with focus on improving sequencing, problem solving, Ⓛ UE strength, and activity tolerance. Calendar will be placed in client's room to increase orientation to month, day, and season. Client's ability to respond to emergency situations will be assessed during next session.

Ryan D, OTR/L

Intervention Plan

Functional Problem Statement #1: *Client needs min to max physical Ⓐ and verbal cues to dress self due to ↓ AROM, activity tolerance, and ability to sequence the task.*
Long-Term Goal #1: *Client will complete all dressing tasks with modified Ⓘ within 2 weeks.*

STG (Objective)	Interventions
STG #1: *Client will don bra with modified Ⓘ using adapted technique within 3 days.*	1. Teach adaptive techniques 2. Post picture of how to don bra by fastening in front. 3. Reinforce correct responses. 4. Teach strengthening program for Ⓛ UE.
STG #2: *Client will don shoes and socks with modified Ⓘ using adapted technique and long shoehorn within 5 days.*	1. Provide long shoe horn and instruct in use. 2. Instruct in adapted techniques for donning shoes and socks. 3. Post picture of adapted technique using long shoe horn. 4. Instruct in use of affected side as a functional assist in dressing. 5. Expand exercise program to include AROM.
STG #3: *Client will complete dressing tasks without verbal cues for sequencing for 3 consecutive days within 10 days.*	1. Verbalize steps before beginning to dress. 2. Verbalize steps while dressing. 3. Post list of steps for client to follow. 4. Take rest breaks as needed for activity tolerance.

Functional Problem Statement #2: *Lack of orientation to environment & inability to problem solve raise safety concerns with ADLs and home management.*
Long-Term Goal #2: *Client will correctly answer questions pertaining to time, date, schedule, and emergency situations using only environmental cues within 2 weeks.*

STG (Objective)	Interventions
STG #1: *Within 1 week, client will correctly identify time, date, and situation without verbal cues when asked on 3 of 3 attempts.*	1. Post calendar, schedule, and emergency information near clock in client's room. 2. Instruct family, nursing staff, and other therapy staff to quiz client several times daily re: date, time, and situation and to reinforce correct responses.

STG #2: Client will follow her daily printed schedule with <2 verbal cues within 1 week.	1. Post daily schedule on wall near clock and review with client during ADL session each morning. 2. Cue client to look at schedule to determine what she should be doing at any given time.
STG #3: Client will correctly problem solve responses to emergency situations Ⓘ on 9 of 10 attempts within 2 weeks.	1. Provide situations for client to problem solve, progressing from easy to more complex. 2. Provide telephone directory or other props as needed for problem solving.

RE-EVALUATION REPORT

In some practice settings, clients must be re-evaluated at certain intervals, such as monthly or quarterly. In other settings, re-evaluation is done as needed. The frequency of re-evaluation depends on the setting, the funding source, and the progress of the client. The tests that were given initially are re-administered, and the results are compared with the results of previous tests to determine the effectiveness of the treatment being provided. The goals and plans are revised at this time and new time lines are projected. Suggested content for this type of report includes the following:

✦ *Client information*: Name/agency, date of birth, gender, applicable medical/educational/developmental diagnoses, precautions, and contraindications

✦ *Occupational profile*: Updates on current areas of occupation that are successful and problematic, contexts and environments that support or hinder occupations, summary of any new medical/education/work information, and updates or changes to client's priorities and targeted outcomes

✦ *Summary and analysis*: Interpretation and summary of data as related to referring concern and comparison of results with previous evaluation results

✦ *Recommendations*: Changes to occupational therapy services, revision or continuation of goals and objectives, frequency of occupational therapy services, and recommendation for referral to other professionals or agencies where applicable

Reprinted with permission from *Guidelines for Documentation of Occupational Therapy* (AOTA, 2008a).

Hand Clinic Re-evaluation Report

Name: Mary M   **DOB**: 5/12/70   **Sex**: F   **Physician**: Dr. Oliver
Primary Dx: Osteoarthritis of Ⓑ CMC joints   **Secondary Dx**: None
Precautions/Contraindications: None   **Date of Referral**: 6/27/2011
Reason for Referral: Client is 1 month post-surgery (LRTI) to the Ⓛ CMC joint and carpal tunnel release.
Date of Initial Evaluation: 7/05/11   **Date of Re-evaluation**: 8/04/11
Funding Source: University insurance

Occupational Profile: *Mary is a 41-year-old Caucasian female who works as an administrative assistant in the English Department at the University. She lives alone in a small, two-story farmhouse 7 miles outside of town. The house is heated with wood that Mary cuts and stacks in the summer. Mary plants a large vegetable garden each year, in addition to holding both a full-time job at the University and a part-time job in a department store. She began experiencing pain in the CMC joints of both hands approximately 3 years ago. She intends to continue her present living arrangement and both of her jobs. She was originally admitted to the outpatient hand clinic on 7/05/11 at 1 month post-surgery for hand rehabilitation following a successful LRTI and a carpal tunnel release. She is being re-evaluated this date (8/04/11) to determine whether further OT services are needed.*

S: *Client initially reported continuous pain at a level of 3/10 and pain on overexertion of the hand at a level of 5/10 in Ⓛ hand, resulting in irritability and difficulty performing bilateral work and daily living tasks, as well as some tasks requiring left hand use. On this date, she reports no continuous pain and pain at a level of 1/10 when typing for more than 45 minutes without rest breaks.*

   Initial ability to engage in work/ADL/IADL tasks (by client report):

   ❖ *Unable to use keyboard with all fingers of Ⓛ hand. Typed with one finger on standard keyboard.*

   ❖ *Unable to grasp cylindrical objects smaller than 1½ inches (broom handle, toothpaste tube) due to ↓ AROM.*

   ❖ *Unable to wear watch or rings on Ⓛ hand due to swelling.*

❖ *Unable to turn door knob with* Ⓛ *hand to enter house when* Ⓡ *hand is full.*

❖ *Unable to lift laundry basket and other items requiring* Ⓑ *UE use. Unable to lift purse or other items needed for IADL tasks with* Ⓛ *hand.*

Current ability to engage in work/ADL/IADL tasks (by client report):

❖ *Able to use new ergonomic keyboard for primary work task using all fingers.*

❖ *Able to sweep floors with a regular broom.*

❖ *Able to fold laundry using* Ⓑ *hands.*

❖ *Able to grasp small items needed for ADL and IADL tasks (toothpaste tube, key, lids) with* Ⓛ *hand, but not at PLOF.*

❖ *Able to turn doorknob with* Ⓛ *hand if door is unlocked.*

❖ *Able to hang clothes on clothesline, including carrying basket and holding garments with* Ⓛ *hand.*

O:

Initial Eval of Client Factors 7/05/11	**Reassessment of Client Factors 8/04/11**
Total active motion of the wrist: 125°	*Total active motion of the wrist: 160°*
Total active motion of the thumb: 110°	*Total active motion of the thumb: 130°*
Grip strength Ⓡ *41#*	*Grip strength* Ⓡ *41#*
Grip strength Ⓛ *15# (37% of* Ⓡ *hand)*	*Grip strength* Ⓛ *22#*
Pinch not tested	*Pinch not tested*
Mild edema at surgery site	*No edema at surgery site*

Client has participated in three 45-minute visits in outpatient hand clinic since admission on 7/05/11. Active and passive range of motion have been performed and taught to client, and home program has been modified as she progressed. Heat has been used, and the client has purchased a home paraffin unit. Electrical stimulation has been used to elicit specific motion and facilitate strengthening of the flexor pollicis longus. A strengthening program has been added to the HEP, and client is able to demonstrate all HEP exercises correctly. Client has received education on the structure and use of the hand, common features of carpometacarpal (CMC) arthritis, ergonomics of the workstation, energy conservation, use of heat for pain relief, and adapted techniques for ADL activities. Client has been given written material covering the same content and reports implementing recommendations into both home and work activities.

A: *Increase in* Ⓛ *grip strength of 7# shows good progress in strength needed to perform functional tasks. Improved thumb AROM (WFL) and wrist AROM (80% of average) now allow client to perform most work and ADL tasks* Ⓘ *in ways that do not damage the joint. Change to an ergonomic keyboard and understanding and correct self-administration of HEP indicate good potential to continue improvement without further OT services.*

P: *Plan to discontinue OT services at this time as results of re-evaluation indicate no further need for OT services unless new problems arise. Client to call hand clinic if questions arise and follow the home program of heat, exercise, and adapted techniques.*

Brad E, OTR/L, CHT

INTERVENTION

OCCUPATIONAL THERAPY SERVICE CONTACTS

Contact, visit, or treatment notes are used to document each visit or each individual OT session. In some situations, contact notes are required in the health record each time a client is seen. In other cases, the OT keeps attendance records, logs, or informal contact notes, which will later be used for the purpose of writing a progress note. Contact notes are also written to document telephone or e-mail contacts and meetings with others regarding the client. Suggested content includes the following:

✦ *Client information*: Name/agency, date of birth, gender, diagnosis, precautions, and contraindications

✦ *Therapy log*: Date, type of contact, names/positions of persons involved, summary or significant information communicated during contacts, client attendance and participation in intervention, reason service is missed, types of interventions used, client's response, environmental or task modification, assistive or adaptive devices used or fabricated, statement of any training education or consultation provided, and the persons present

Reprinted with permission from *Guidelines for Documentation of Occupational Therapy* (AOTA, 2008a).

Acute Care Unit Contact Note

Client: Curt G   **Sex**: M   **DOB**: 9/12/49   **Health Record #**: 123456
Dx: Guillain-Barré syndrome   **Physician**: Dr. McDonald
Date: 4/14/11   **Time**: 8:30 AM

S: Pt. reports, "I want to get out of this bed. It's been a long night."

O: Client participated in bedside OT session in ICU for instruction in ADL tasks and AROM in Ⓑ UEs. Client required mod Ⓐ supine → sit. Upon sitting, O_2 saturation dropped to ~85%. Grooming, dressing, and UE AROM activities not completed due to low O_2 levels. Client returned to supine with min Ⓐ. After ~2 minutes, O_2 levels returned to ~95%. Client washed face $\bar{p}$ set-up in supine but declined further activity, citing fatigue. ICU nurse was notified of pt's change in O_2 saturation during activity.

A: Ability to transition supine to sit indicates improved activity tolerance from yesterday when pt was unable to tolerate this. Expressed interest for out-of-bed activity is a good indication for improving strength and function. Decreased activity tolerance related to drop in O_2 saturation with exertion limits ability to participate in self-care tasks. Client would benefit from instruction in energy conservation as well as correct positioning to ↓ exertion and ↑ activity tolerance for ADL tasks. At this time, pt does not have the ability to tolerate 3 hours daily therapy required for rehab unit stay; however, pt would benefit from continued therapy at SNF level once medically stable.

P: Continue skilled OT daily to ↑ activity tolerance and Ⓘ in ADL tasks for 5 days or until discharge from acute care.

Abbie B, OTR/L

Outpatient Clinic Contact Note

Client: Makayla L   **Sex**: F   **DOB**: 6/16/07   **Health Record #**: 123456
Dx: Spina bifida   **Physician**: Dr. Wright   **Date**: 8/19/11

Received phone call from child's mother canceling today's appointment due to schedule conflict. Mother was reminded of clinic attendance policy as child has now missed 3 of last 5 scheduled weekly appointments; mother voiced understanding that one more missed appointment may result in Makayla being discharged from OT services. Offered to change OT appointment to a more convenient time for family, mother declined this offer. Also reminded mother of 6-month meeting with therapy team and service coordinator from County Agency that is scheduled for 8/24/11; mother reports plan to attend that meeting and next OT visit on 8/26/11.

Nicki W, OTR/L

PROGRESS REPORT

Progress notes are written on a regularly scheduled basis (usually weekly or monthly), with the time frame determined by the facility. The facility is guided by accrediting agencies and funding sources in determining the time frame in which progress notes must be written. The progress note provides a summary of the intervention process and documents the client's progress toward goals. It also includes recommendations for continuation/discontinuation of services and referral to other health care professionals if appropriate. Suggested content includes the following:

+ *Client information*: Name/agency, date of birth, gender, diagnosis, precautions, and contraindication
+ *Summary of services provided*: Brief statement about the frequency of services and length of time services have been provided; techniques and strategies used; environmental or task modifications provided; adaptive equipment or orthotics provided; medical, educational, or other pertinent client updates; client's response to occupational therapy services; and programs or training provided to the client or caregivers
+ *Current client performance*: Client's progress toward the goals and client's performance in areas of occupations
+ *Plan or recommendations*: Recommendations and rationale as well as client's input to changes or continuation of plan

Reprinted with permission from *Guidelines for Documentation of Occupational Therapy* (AOTA, 2008a).

Behavioral Health Center Progress Note

Client: Erica H   *Sex*: F   *DOB*: 10/12/69   *Health Record #*: 123456
Dx: Depression   *Physician*: Dr. Stephens   *Date*: 8/19/11

S: *In assertion group on 8/17/11, client talked about how her life had taken a "downward spiral" since early July, and she had become more passive and less proactive in getting her needs met, although she had not been aware of it at the time.*

O: *Client attended assertion group 2/2, communication group 1/1, and IADL group 3/5 this week. She was on time to 4/6 groups without reminders, wearing neatly pressed clothing, makeup, and hair clips. In assertion group on 8/17, she shared without prompting 2 stories about her usual way of dealing with retail situations. In communication group, she spontaneously answered one question addressed to the group as a whole, and in IADL group, she offered to assist another client with his checkbook.*

A: *Client's spontaneous actions in groups and willingness to share verbally indicate an improved mood this week. Group attendance for 6/8 groups is much improved this week as compared to 2/8 group attendance last week. Improved dress, hygiene, and makeup also indicate an improved mood from last week. Client would benefit from planning a structure for her days to prevent another "downward spiral" after discharge.*
  Goals #1 (assertion) and #2 (communication) are met as of this date.
  Goal #3 (leisure skills) is continued through discharge on 8/20/11 pending formulation of a plan.
  Goal #4 (parenting skills) was discontinued on 8/15/11.

P: *Client to be seen in IADL group for 1 more day, with discharge anticipated tomorrow afternoon 8/20/11. IADL group will be used for preparing the structured plan for using her time. Will meet with client individually if needed to ensure that written plan is completed.*
Stephanie A, OTR/L

TRANSITION PLAN

A transition plan is written whenever a client transfers from one setting to another within a service delivery system. It is designed to provide client information to the new service provider so that care is uninterrupted. Transition plans summarize the client's current occupational status, specify what service setting the client is leaving, state what setting the client is entering, and tell how and when the transition will occur. Suggested content includes the following:

- *Client information*: Name/agency, date of birth, gender, diagnosis, precautions, and contraindications
- *Client's current status*: Client's current performance in occupations
- *Transition plan*: Name of current service setting and name of setting to which client will transition, reason for transition, time frame in which transition will occur, and outline of activities to be carried out during the transition plan
- *Recommendations*: Recommendations and rationale for occupational therapy services, modification or accommodations needed, and assistive technology and environmental modification needed

Reprinted with permission from *Guidelines for Documentation of Occupational Therapy* (AOTA, 2008a).

Transition Plan

Name: Keonna W   *DOB*: 4/29/08   *Gender*: Female
Date of Plan: 4/11/11   *Expected Transition Date*: May 2011
Diagnosis: TBI, s/p MVA   *Precautions*: Seizure disorder

Occupational History: *Keonna experienced head and multiple orthopedic injuries following a MVA at 9 days of age. Since that time, she has had multiple cranial, hip, and leg surgeries. She is currently under the management of a neurologist as well as an orthopedist. The mother carries out a home program daily, which is designed to stimulate development.*

S: *The mother reports that although Keonna's seizures, multiple surgeries, and illnesses have slowed her development, the family is hopeful that Keonna will progress more rapidly through her developmental milestones now that the surgeries are finished and the seizures are under control.*

O: *Child received her first OT screening in the hospital 1 week post-injury. She received formal developmental assessments at 2, 4, 6, 12, and 24 months of age. Parents were given home program following the initial formal* *assessment. OT sessions were started twice weekly at 12 months of age and have continued to this date; Keonna has also been followed every 3 months in the Birth-to-Three Developmental Clinic. She is now eligible for preschool services as she will be turning 3 later this month.*

Current occupational performance: *Current problems being treated in OT include visual regard and visually directed reach, midline orientation, postural symmetry, and motor overflow. Current goals for Keonna include functional reach, grasp and release, rolling, and ability to sustain antigravity positions for ADLs and developmental play activities. Keonna requires an adaptive chair to maintain upright positioning. She is dependent in all self-care tasks, including feeding. She requires hand over hand assistance to initiate play with toys.*

A: *Keonna's current skills indicate functioning at about a 4-month level of development. Although the mother provides a stimulating environment, Keonna would benefit from continuation of regular OT, PT, and speech therapy services to facilitate her continued progress through the developmental sequence.*

P: *Keonna will receive her first preschool service evaluation next month in May 2011. Parents have been given a home program, which has been updated as child has progressed in treatment. Home program will continue through the transition to preschool services.*

David W, OTS

Alicia L, OTR/L (co-signature of a student's note by the supervising therapist)

OUTCOMES

DISCHARGE REPORT—SUMMARY OF OT SERVICES AND OUTCOMES

A discharge summary (also called a *discontinuation report*) is used to summarize the changes in the client's ability to engage in occupation and to make recommendations for referral or follow-up care if needed. Discharge notes often follow a format of their own, stating the date and purpose of the referral and giving a summary of the initial findings, the course of treatment, a summary of progress, and any recommendations for follow-up care. Discharge summaries may be done as SOAP or narrative notes, or the facility may have a particular form that is used. Some facilities use the same form for evaluation, re-evaluation, and discharge, making it quicker to prepare the discontinuation report. Suggested content includes the following:

✦ *Client information*: Name/agency, date of birth, gender, diagnosis, precautions, and contraindications

✦ *Summary of intervention process*: Date of initial and final service; frequency, number of sessions, summary of interventions used; summary of progress toward goals; and occupational therapy outcomes—initial client status and ending status regarding engagement in occupations, client's assessment of efficacy of occupational therapy services

✦ *Recommendations*: Recommendations pertaining to the client's future needs; specific follow-up plans, if applicable; and referrals to other professionals and agencies, if applicable

Reprinted with permission from *Guidelines for Documentation of Occupational Therapy* (AOTA, 2008a).

Occupational Therapy Discharge Summary

Name: *Ruby C*   **DOB**: *4/10/40*   **Dx**: Ⓛ *SDH*
Physician: *Dr. Armin*   **Date**: *2/19/11*

S: *Client reports that she is very pleased with the outcome of her OT treatment, and with her ability to take care of herself at home. She reports no steps to the front entrance of a one-story home, and no architectural barriers inside the house. She reports that she owns the following adaptive equipment already: wheeled walker, reacher, dressing stick, sock aide, long shoehorn, tub bench, raised toilet seat, and grab board around the toilet and in the tub/shower.*

O: *Client participated in 20/20 OT sessions bedside and in OT clinic from SOC on 2/06/11.*

ADL Status on 2/06/11	**ADL Status on 2/19/11**
Mod Ⓐ *in transfers*	*SBA in transfers*
Mod Ⓐ *in toileting*	Ⓘ *in toileting*
Mod Ⓐ *in feeding*	*SBA in feeding after set-up*
Mod Ⓐ *in dressing*	*Dressing from arm chair requires set-up and SBA for standing to pull up pants.*
Max Ⓐ *for safety in bathing*	*SBA for bathing with min* Ⓐ *w/c* ↔ *shower using tub bench*

Client education provided in adaptive equipment techniques and HEP; client demonstrated ability to perform correctly. Home modifications were discussed with client and caregiver.

A: *Differences in admission and discharge abilities for ADLs show good progress. Since caregiver is available to provide SBA needed for safety in ADL tasks, all treatment goals have been met, and client is ready for discharge.*

P: *Client will be discharged home tomorrow. Client to continue home exercise program. Adaptive equipment recommended: walker basket and reacher holder for walker. Client and caregiver to decide how to implement home modifications. Client will continue with outpatient physical therapy. No direct occupational therapy services are recommended at this time.*

Anya A, OTR/L

Now let us consider the same note, written on a form provided by the rehabilitation facility:

Rehabilitation Center—OT Discharge Note

Name: *Ruby C*   **DOB:** *4/10/40*   **Dx:** Ⓛ *SDH*
Physician: *Dr. Armin*   **Date:** *2/19/11*

Course of Rehabilitation: *Client participated in 20/20 session from SOC on 2/06/11. Skilled instruction in adaptive techniques for ADLs provided. Client progress was good and she met all tx. goals. Client now requires SBA in all transfers, lower body ADLs, upper body ADLs, grooming/hygiene. She is Ⓘ in toileting. Client also requires SBA in feeding after set-up. Client completes dressing from arm chair with wheeled walker, set-up, and SBA for standing to pull pants over hips. Bathing is SBA with min Ⓐ w/c ↔ shower using tub bench.*

Client Education: *Recommendations for additional adaptive equipment and modifications to home discussed with client and caregiver. Client and caregiver were instructed in home exercise program of theraband, free weights, wands, and other activities to choose from for Ⓑ UE strengthening. Client demonstrated ability to perform exercises correctly.*

Discharge Recommendations/Referrals: *Discharge home with caregiver. Continue home exercise program. Adaptive equipment recommended: walker basket and reacher holder for walker. Client already has wheeled walker, reacher, dressing stick, sock aide, long shoehorn, and functional bathroom equipment and has demonstrated ability to use these correctly and safely. Client will be seen in outpatient PT. No direct OT services are recommended at this time.*

Anya A, OTR/L

14

Documentation in Different Practice Settings

In this chapter, we will examine documentation in several different practice situations. Each of these practice settings has some requirements that are specific to the setting or the primary payment source. Documentation in these settings is different in some ways from the examples you have learned so far.

DOCUMENTATION IN MENTAL HEALTH

If you go from a job in a rehabilitation center to one in a mental health setting, you might think that nothing you have learned about documentation applies. Problems, goals, and interventions are often multidisciplinary and may be written in a different format from what you have learned. The language used in the documentation may seem less specific. Some mental health issues, such as suicide risk or past sexual abuse, may not fit very neatly into the *Framework-II* (AOTA, 2008b; Holmquist, 2004). Also, intervention is often provided in groups or within a therapeutic environment or milieu. OT services may be included in a treatment service designated as adjunctive therapy, activity therapy, or expressive therapy, which may include therapeutic recreation specialists, music therapists, art therapists, and dance therapists. Professional roles often overlap and there is often a blurring of professional identities. Reimbursement may not be discipline-specific and therapy services may be included in the room rate for the facility.

One of the exceptions is geriatric psychiatric mental health units or partial hospitalization units where services are reimbursed through Medicare. With Medicare reimbursement, documentation is similar to inpatient Medicare requirements, but the types of intervention covered include psychiatric OT services as well as self-care interventions (Roberts & Evenson, 2009).

Psychosocial interventions are at the very root of OT and are still fundamental to OT practice as a whole (AOTA, 2010b). From its inception to the present, OT has been holistic and client-centered. OT in mental health is based "in the belief in the therapeutic value of meaningful occupation and the importance of satisfying interpersonal relationships and balance in the daily routines of work, self-care, and leisure" (Paterson, 2008, p. 14). Whether in a rehabilitation center or in a mental health setting, the attention to psychosocial aspects of a client's life is critical to the ability to resume engagement in meaningful areas of occupation (AOTA, 2010b). Client-centered OT means collaborating with the client throughout the OT process to maximize engagement in meaningful areas of occupation (Rosa, 2009). Nowhere is this more important than in psychosocial practice settings, where clients come to us with serious disruptions in their ability to engage in meaningful occupations.

INITIAL EVALUATION REPORTS

While you may be contributing to a multidisciplinary initial evaluation, it is essential to obtain a comprehensive occupational profile from which to plan interventions. This may be achieved through an informal interview or by using one of the many standardized occupational performance measures that are available (Hemphill-Pearson, 2008). The occupational profile will highlight the areas of occupation that are dysfunctional or interrupted and provide information about the context(s) to which the client will return.

Gateley CA, Borcherding S. *Documentation Manual for Occupational Therapy: Writing SOAP Notes, 3rd Edition* (pp. 169-188)
© 2012 SLACK Incorporated

FUNCTIONAL PROBLEM STATEMENTS

Functional problem statements in a mental health practice setting are traditionally divided into two parts. The problem itself is stated in one or two words, such as *chemical dependence, noncompliant behavior,* or *suicide risk.* The behavioral manifestations that follow define the areas of occupation and the contributing factors involved.

Problem: Chemical dependence
Behavioral Manifestations: *Mark has been using alcohol since age 12, with increasing frequency over the past year, and also admits to using cocaine, crystal meth, opium, and marijuana, resulting in a failed marriage, loss of two jobs, and involvement with the criminal justice system.*

Problem: Noncompliant behavior
Behavioral Manifestations: *Client disobeys foster parents by running away, refusing to follow rules or requests, and engaging in sexual activity, resulting in six foster home placements in the past 4 years.*

Problem: Suicide risk
Behavioral Manifestations: *During the week prior to admission, the client verbalized suicidal ideation, stating that life was no longer worth living. On the day of admission he purchased a handgun.*

Problem: Increased voices
Behavioral Manifestations: *For two weeks prior to admission, client reported that he was hearing more voices. Client reports that the voices made it difficult for him to concentrate, and staff at his group home described him as becoming more irritable.*

INTERVENTION PLANS

Intervention plans in mental health are usually multidisciplinary. The "therapeutic milieu," or the total environment of the setting, is often considered to be critical in caring for clients who have mental health disorders. The individualized treatment plan (ITP) in a mental health setting is a contract for change between the client and the treatment team. Ideally, after each individual discipline assesses the client's needs and strengths, each individual discipline suggests goals, objectives, and interventions for treatment within that discipline. All goals, objectives, and interventions for each discipline involved in the client's care are then written into one comprehensive plan. Major problems or concerns identified in the evaluation are documented on the ITP. The client is a participant in the intervention process and signs the treatment plan to show agreement with it. These plans are similar to those developed by teams in a rehabilitation or school setting but differ in that all clinicians work toward the same goals through different interventions.

Success in writing a multidisciplinary treatment plan depends on the following:

✦ The involvement of the client (and family, if they are currently involved in the client's life).

✦ The willingness of each member of the treatment team to cooperate in a coordinated effort to effect change.

✦ Regular evaluation of the effectiveness of the plan and changes in direction in interventions that have not been effective.

In actual practice, however, the length of stay is sometimes so brief that a client may be discharged before a comprehensive evaluation plan can be formalized.

INTERVENTION STRATEGIES

Occupational therapists use a wide variety of interventions in psychosocial settings to promote empowerment and facilitate personal change, including the following:

✦ Modification of the environment

✦ Reintegration into the community

✦ Motivational interviewing

✦ Cognitive behavioral approaches

While the goal of occupational therapy in mental health is improved engagement in areas of occupation, the interventions often target specific performance skills, such as the following:

✦ Assertiveness

✦ Problem solving

✦ Self-awareness

+ Anger management
+ Sequencing
+ Prioritizing
+ Role identification and development
+ Communication and social skills (AOTA, 2008b; Creek, 2008)

Occupational therapy interventions focus on the occupations that are disrupted or that the client would like to pursue in the future. Ideally, the documentation of services provided in psychosocial programs reflects the occupation-based approach of our profession. This means that your documentation should be objective, measurable, and focused on the client's occupational profile and ability to engage in necessary and valued life activities.

Interventions may be specific to occupational therapy, or they may be broader and applicable to activity therapy. The choice of interventions may depend largely upon what treatment groups are being provided by the facility, with the ability to individualize intervention strategies within the groups themselves. Selecting meaningful treatment interventions can be an interesting challenge. For example, most clients may attend communication groups, but within those groups, you will customize the way you choose to increase communication skills for each individual client. With a little experience, you will learn to individualize goals for each client in the group, while still providing for the needs of the group as a whole.

When planning intervention strategies, the client's assets (good verbal skills, intelligence, etc.) will be the tools that the client has to use in overcoming his or her problems. A "strength" in this context is an ability, a skill, or an interest that the client has used in the past or has the potential for using. Assets can include such things as the client's interests (enjoys playing music), abilities (writes well), relationship skills (has a good relationship with her father), and social support systems (minister keeps in contact). Assets may also be past abilities that the treatment team wants to encourage as treatment progresses (Jane was physically active before she became ill). Some interests (enjoys going to bars on weekends) may not be assets.

CONTACT AND PROGRESS NOTES

The use of contact and progress notes may vary by facility. Some of the exceptions are geriatric psychiatric inpatient and partial hospitalization units where the clients are insured through Medicare. In these settings, the documentation follows Medicare requirements.

If a client with a mental health diagnosis is seen in home health, the Medicare standards for home health apply, with a treatment note required for each visit. In long-term psychiatric facilities, where progress notes rather than treatment notes are used, the therapist keeps a log of attendance and makes notes about participation and behaviors that show progress each day, and then compiles that information into a progress note in the health record at regular intervals. In acute care psychiatric facilities, where length of stay may be just a few days, notes may be written for each group the client attends in order to reflect the client's progress from day to day.

When you begin thinking in the language of mental health, terms like *brightened affect, less delusional,* or *improved mood* begin to enter your vocabulary, and you may be tempted to write in less objective and measurable terms. However, there are observable behavioral manifestations that help you determine that the client's affect is brighter or his mood is improved. Perhaps you are seeing him smile more frequently, initiate conversation more often, or respond to your "hello" by making eye contact. Perhaps the client's comments had less delusional content and were directly related to the topic discussed in group. Perhaps she takes less time to get up and dress in the morning or is more easily persuaded to attend OT. These indicators are all measurable, and it is very helpful to the treatment team if you are able to report your observations in measurable and behavioral terms.

The trend toward role diffusion is making it more difficult to document occupational therapy as a service that offers good value for the dollars spent in mental health care. As resources shrink and costs expand, we need to focus on documenting functional changes that are cost-effective and meaningful to both the payer and to the consumer. There are myriad factors present in the lives of people with serious mental illness and chemical dependency that hinder their ability to engage in meaningful occupations. In a situation where so much role diffusion is present, occupational therapists need to be **clear** and **specific** about the way our services facilitate "positive outcomes such as improvements in sensorimotor, cognitive, and psychosocial abilities, which all contribute to overall health, well-being, and life satisfaction" (Mathieson & Hahn, 2010, p. 10).

CRITICAL CARE PATHWAYS IN MENTAL HEALTH

As length of stay has shortened for psychiatric diagnoses, some mental health settings have begun using critical care pathways and computer-generated intervention plans for the most common problems seen in that setting.

These are time savers and can be customized to the client by adding desired outcomes and treatment interventions specific to the individual client.

Critical care pathways in mental health are multidisciplinary and are conceptually the same as those in rehabilitation. The plan for the client's care each day for each discipline is preplanned in order to make the most efficient use of staff time during the short length of stay, while still making sure the client's needs are met.

COMPUTER-GENERATED PLANS

In an electronic "mix-and-match" program, the computer provides prompts from which the team or the individual therapist selects the problem statements, goals, objectives, and treatment interventions that will be used for the individual client. When using prepackaged treatment planning sheets, the problems are expressed briefly (e.g., *depressed mood, drug abuse, suicide risk*), and the behavioral manifestations that apply to the individual client are written in.

There is a list of long-term goals, or **outcomes**, such as:

✦ *Within 1 week, the client will identify 3 new coping strategies to use when he feels the urge to use drugs.*

✦ *Within 1 week, the client will identify 2 social or leisure activities that do not involve the use of drugs or alcohol.*

The treatment team chooses goals for each client who is admitted. All members of the interdisciplinary treatment team work on these goals during the client's hospital stay. On a computer generated form, there is also a list of potential interventions that would be addressed by the treatment team. Interventions might include strategies such as:

✦ *Evaluate the client.*

✦ *Encourage client to express emotions.*

✦ *Teach new coping skills.*

✦ *Encourage the client to verbalize alternatives to previous coping strategies.*

✦ *Assist the client to develop a discharge plan that will prevent recurrence.*

Interventions are chosen for use with each client. Each discipline implements the interventions in its own way. In relation to the five intervention strategies listed above, you might:

✦ Do an occupational profile to determine specific problems in each area of occupation.

✦ Use OT media to encourage the client to express emotions.

✦ Use OT groups to teach new coping skills and to help the client find alternatives to strategies that have not worked well in the past.

✦ Help the client make a plan for any areas of occupation that were part of the previous problem.

Social work adapts the same treatment interventions to individual and group therapy, and nursing implements the interventions on the unit. In this situation, there are sheets provided for each goal that is commonly used. The interventions are individualized to the client by stating behavioral manifestations of the problem and by adding and deleting outcomes and/or interventions. An example of such a prepackaged treatment planning sheet for alcohol dependence follows on the next page. It is provided only as an example of what might be seen in practice. Please note that the desired outcomes may not meet the COAST criteria you have learned since they are general outcomes to be addressed by the multidisciplinary treatment team.

In Chapter 12, we considered treatment interventions for Heather, a psychiatric client admitted after a suicide attempt. If a treatment team were using computer-generated planning for Heather's care, the first step would be to go to the computer and pull up multidisciplinary treatment planning sheets. For Heather, some of the choices might be:

✦ Suicide attempt

✦ Poor concentration

✦ Anger

✦ Poor self-esteem

On each sheet there would be a place to identify Heather's behavior in relation to the problem. Following that might be a list of interventions commonly used for that problem, starting with evaluation and ending with discharge planning. Interventions that really do not apply to Heather would be deleted, and any additional interventions that apply to her uniquely would be added. The groups provided by the facility would be listed as interventions and you would plan for ways to make OT groups offered daily meet Heather's needs. There would be a list of desired outcomes for each of Heather's identified problems, with a place to add outcomes specific to Heather's situation.

BEHAVIORAL HEALTH MULTIDISCIPLINARY TREATMENT PLAN

Client Name: **Date:**

Problem #:   **Problem Name:** Alcohol dependence

Behavioral Manifestations:

Desired Outcomes	Target Date	Date Achieved
1. Client will verbally acknowledge that alcohol use has been a problem and will state intent to abstain from alcohol use.		
2. Client will have developed at least three new ways to deal with stress and will have demonstrated use of these.		
3. Client will have an aftercare plan in place.		
4. Client will have established a 5-day period of sobriety and of attending AA meetings daily.		
5.		
6.		

Treatment Interventions	Staff Responsible
1. Evaluation of the client's alcohol intake and use patterns.	
2. Provide individual, group, and family therapy.	
3. Education re: the disease model of chemical dependency.	
4. Provide opportunities to express feelings.	
5. Teach coping skills.	
6. Assist client to restructure environmental situations.	
7. Evaluate and teach relationship skills.	
8. Facilitate peer confrontation and feedback.	
9. Introduce social/leisure activities that do not include alcohol.	
10. Develop plan with client on how to respond when experiencing cravings for alcohol.	
11.	

I agree with this plan.

_____

Client's signature

Documentation in School-Based Practice

If you provide OT services in a school setting, your documentation will be related to the child's Individualized Education Program (IEP). The IEP is a written document that details a student's educational and functional needs (Jackson, 2007; U.S. Department of Education, 2006). In other OT practice settings, OTs write a specific intervention plan. In school-based practice, the IEP serves as the intervention plan. The *Individuals With Disabilities Education Act* (IDEA) was re-authorized in 2004 and established the following requirements for content of an IEP:

✦ A statement of the child's present level of academic achievement and functional performance

✦ A statement of measurable annual goals, including academic and functional goals that enable the child to participate and progress in the general education curriculum

✦ A description of benchmarks or short-term objectives for children who take alternate assessments to measure achievement standards

✦ A description of how the child's progress toward annual goals will be measured and reported upon

✦ A statement of the special education and related services to be provided to the child

✦ A statement of individual accommodations to measure the academic achievement and functional performance of the child on state and district assessments (U.S. Department of Education, 2010, p. 1)

The U.S. Department of Education provides an example of a model IEP form at http://idea.ed.gov. Most states also have model forms that combine the federal requirements with specific state requirements. Regardless of the specific format used by a particular state or district, OT is considered a "related service" as described in the requirements above. The IEP is developed by a team consisting of the child's parents, regular education teacher(s), special education teacher(s), and related services personnel (Bazyk & Case-Smith, 2010). Rather than writing separate OT goals, the OT should contribute to the development of the overall IEP, including annual goals "which the OT may support or address as a related service" (Chandler, 2007, p. 16).

Since an IEP can be quite lengthy, the one provided here has been condensed to show only the aspects that are most pertinent to OT.

Individualized Education Program

Name: Truman T   *Date of Birth:* 7/24/2005   *Age:* 5 yrs, 11 mos
School Year: 2011-2012   *Grade Level:* Kindergarten
IEP Meeting Date: 7/22/2011   *IEP Initiation/Duration Dates:* 8/8/11 to 5/26/12

Present Level of Academic Achievement and Functional Performance

Truman will be six years old in just a few days. He was diagnosed with Pervasive Developmental Disorder (PDD) at age two. He attended the Early Childhood Special Education program for two years during the 2008-2009 and 2009-2010 school years and Kindergarten during the 2010-2011 school year. The decision has been made by the IEP team to retain Truman in Kindergarten for the upcoming 2011-2012 school year. Truman's parents are in agreement with this decision and hope that another year in Kindergarten will allow him to improve his academic performance and social skills prior to advancing to 1st grade. Truman does not qualify for Extended School Year services at this time.

Truman spends the majority of his day in the general education classroom with a paraprofessional present for support with classroom participation. He spends 60 minutes daily in the special education classroom for additional 1:1 and small group instruction in reading and writing skills. He also participates in adaptive physical education twice weekly for 45 minutes.

Truman's verbal skills are delayed in comparison to same-age peers, although he has demonstrated considerable improvement over the past year. He is now able to communicate in three- to five-word sentences consistently. He also utilizes a Picture Exchange Communication System (PECS) to supplement his verbal communication.

Truman is easily distracted by auditory and visual stimuli in and near the classroom and has difficulty remaining in his seat for more than 5 minutes at a time. He has difficulty with transitions between activities and locations, but this has improved following implementation of a visual schedule. Truman sometimes responds with negative behaviors (yelling, hitting, pinching) when classmates inadvertently touch or bump into him during classroom activities.

Truman is hesitant to engage in play activities with his peers. He prefers to play alone and does not initiate interactions with peers. Toward the end of last school year, he was beginning to participate in some simple ball activities with others during recess with significant support from his paraprofessional. He will continue participation in a weekly after-school peer communication group led by the elementary school counselor.

Truman is able to recognize all letters of the alphabet, but he does not yet read any words. He can copy the letters of his name when provided with a visual model, but legibility is inconsistent. His ability to copy other letters of the alphabet remains very inconsistent. Truman has difficulty achieving a tripod grasp on writing utensils and staying on the lines of standard writing paper. He also has difficulty with consistent letter size and spacing. His writing performance improves with the use of adaptive writing paper and rubber pencil grip. He does consistently copy basic shapes including circle, square, triangle, and cross.

Truman requires assistance to obtain and carry his tray in the lunchroom. He is easily upset by the noise in the lunchroom and often needs to be taken to a quieter room to finish lunch. Truman consistently indicates when he needs to use the restroom, but continues to have difficulty managing the button and zipper on his jeans. He needs hand-over-hand assistance to complete hand washing because he prefers to play in the water. Truman is now able to take his coat on and off independently. He can also manage Velcro tennis shoes independently.

Type of Service	*Anticipated Frequency*	*Amount of Time*	*Location of Service*
Special Education *Special education teacher will provide intensive reading and writing instruction in both 1:1 and small group formats.*	*Daily*	*60 minutes*	*Special Education Classroom*
Supplementary Aids & Services *Truman will have a paraprofessional present throughout the school day except when with the special education teacher.*	*Daily*	*340 minutes*	*General Education Classroom & Across Settings*
Program Modifications *Adaptive P.E.*	*Weekly*	*90 minutes*	*Indoor/Outdoor P.E. Settings*
Accommodations for Assessments *Truman will be allowed additional time for completion of classroom and state assessments.*	*Weekly*	*60 minutes*	*General and Special Education Classrooms*
Related Services *Occupational Therapy*	*Weekly*	*30 minutes*	*General and Special Education Classrooms & Across Settings*
Related Services *Speech Language Pathology*	*Weekly*	*90 minutes*	*General and Special Education Classrooms & Across Settings*

Annual Goal #1: *Using compensatory strategies, Truman will demonstrate legible handwriting in the classroom with appropriate baseline orientation, letter size, and spacing with 80% accuracy on 4 of 5 consecutive days.*

Evaluation Methods:
☐ *Curriculum-Based Assessment*
☐ *State Assessments*
☑ *Data Collection Chart*
☑ *Work Samples*
☐ *Other:*

Primary Implementers:
☑ *General Education Teacher*
☑ *Special Education Teacher*
☐ *Physical Therapy*
☑ *Occupational Therapy*
☐ *Speech Language Pathology*
☐ *Other:*

Measurable Benchmarks/Objectives:
1. *Truman will demonstrate tripod grasp on writing utensils using adaptive pencil grip with 80% accuracy on 4 of 5 consecutive days.*
2. *Truman will write his first name on adaptive paper without a visual model, demonstrating appropriate letter formation, size, and line orientation on 4 of 5 consecutive days.*
3. *Truman will copy 22/26 lowercase letters onto adaptive paper using a visual model, demonstrating appropriate letter formation, size, and line orientation on 4 of 5 consecutive days.*

Date of Mastery:
1.

2.

3.

Annual Goal #2: Truman will demonstrate improved attention and work behaviors during classroom activities with no more than three sensory breaks per hour throughout the day on 4 of 5 consecutive days.	
Evaluation Methods: ☐ Curriculum-Based Assessment ☐ State Assessments ☑ Data Collection Chart ☐ Work Samples ☐ Other:	**Primary Implementers:** ☑ General Education Teacher ☑ Special Education Teacher ☐ Physical Therapy ☑ Occupational Therapy ☐ Speech Language Pathology ☐ Other:
Measurable Benchmarks/Objectives: 1. Truman will remain seated at his desk or during circle time for 15 minutes with minimal verbal cues and no more than one sensory break. 2. Truman will transition between classroom activities with minimal verbal cues using a visual schedule and without demonstrating negative behaviors (yelling, hitting, etc.) toward peers and staff with 80% accuracy on 4 of 5 consecutive days. 3. Truman will tolerate unexpected touch from classmates without demonstrating negative behaviors (yelling, hitting, etc.) with 80% accuracy on 4 of 5 consecutive days.	**Date of Mastery:** 1. 2. 3.

Annual Goal #3: Truman will demonstrate school-related self-care skills with no more than minimal assistance using adaptive strategies with 80% accuracy on 4 of 5 consecutive days.	
Evaluation Methods: ☐ Curriculum-Based Assessment ☐ State Assessments ☑ Data Collection Chart ☐ Work Samples ☐ Other:	**Primary Implementers:** ☐ General Education Teacher ☐ Special Education Teacher ☐ Physical Therapy ☑ Occupational Therapy ☐ Speech Language Pathology ☑ Other: Paraprofessional
Measurable Benchmarks/Objectives: 1. Truman will complete toileting without assistance to manage clothing fasteners with 80% accuracy on 4 of 5 consecutive days. 2. Truman will wash hands following a visual schedule with minimal verbal cues with 80% accuracy on 4 of 5 consecutive days. 3. Truman will obtain/transport his lunch tray and remain seated in the cafeteria for the duration of the lunch period with minimal verbal cues on 4 of 5 consecutive days.	**Date of Mastery:** 1. 2. 3.

DOCUMENTATION IN SKILLED NURSING FACILITIES IN LONG-TERM CARE

Most clients who receive therapy services in skilled nursing facilities in long-term settings are covered by Medicare, and documentation may be done using specialized Medicare forms. When a client is first admitted, a multidisciplinary evaluation called the Minimum Data Set (MDS) is used to determine the specific level of care needed. The MDS is part of the federally mandated process for clinical assessment of residents in Medicare and Medicaid certified long-term care facilities (CMS, 2010b). You can view this form and instructions on how to complete it at the CMS Web site at www.cms.gov/CMSForms. For ease and efficiency, each discipline may be assigned a specific part of the MDS to complete. Facilities may vary in how ADLs, cognitive, or other sections are divided between OT, nursing, or other disciplines. Facilities will also vary in terms of other formats for OT-specific documentation.

Documentation in Outpatient Settings

Documentation requirements in outpatient settings will depend on the facility requirements, accrediting agencies, and funding sources. Managed care insurance may require a special form that outlines the client's evaluation results and plan of care before additional visits will be approved. This form is in addition to the facility evaluation form that must be completed.

For outpatient clients who have Medicare as a funding source, the occupational therapy initial assessment may be recorded on a CMS 700 form (Figure 14-1), and progress notes may be recorded on a CMS 701 form (Figure 14-2). These forms and instructions on how to complete them are available at www.cms.gov/CMSForms. CMS does not require the use of these forms as long as all required information is present on the facility form (American Physical Therapy Association [APTA], 2010). As you can see in the examples, these forms have very limited space available for recording data.

Documentation in an Inpatient Rehabilitation Facility

Clients admitted to an inpatient rehabilitation facility will have an interdisciplinary evaluation documented on a tool called the Inpatient Rehabilitation Facility Patient Assessment Instrument (IRF-PAI), available at www.cms.gov/InpatientRehabFacPPS/04_IRFPAI.asp. While there likely will be separate supporting documentation required in a specific facility format, the OT contributes to the IRF-PAI by providing information about the client's Functional Independence Measure (FIM) scores. As explained in Chapter 3, the FIM instrument measures the client's level of independence in 18 functional activities in the categories of self-care, sphincter control, transfers, locomotion, communication, and social cognition (UDSMR, 2010). FIM scores for each area are documented at admission. FIM score goals are then set and tracked at regular intervals (typically weekly), and then FIM scores are again recorded at the time of discharge. Documentation in the OT initial evaluation, contact/progress notes, and discharge summary should include information specific to the functional activities scored by the FIM instrument.

Documentation in Early Intervention

Children receiving OT as part of federally mandated early intervention services will have a document called the Individualized Family Service Plan (IFSP). While each state will have a specific format for the IFSP, there are certain elements that must be contained in the document, such as the following:

+ Present level in the areas of physical, cognitive, communication, social, emotional, and adaptive (self-care) development
+ Family's resources, priorities, and concerns for the child
+ Expected outcomes for the child and family
+ Specific early intervention services needed
+ Natural environments in which services will be provided
+ Dates of initiation and anticipated duration of services
+ Name of service coordinator
+ Plan for transition to preschool or other services at age 3 (Pape & Ryba, 2004)

A unique feature of early intervention services is that all documentation is written in plain language that is understandable to parents rather than in professional jargon. While SOAP note format is not used, you can see that all of the SOAP elements are still included:

Desiree participated in a 30-minute OT session in her home with her mother and grandmother present. Focus this date was on self-feeding. Mother reports that Desiree has been feeding herself finger foods from the highchair tray but is not showing much interest in using a spoon. With Desiree seated in the highchair, mother showed how she helps her hold the spoon to scoop yogurt out of the container, but Desiree became fussy and threw the spoon down. Suggestion was made to place yogurt in small bowl to make scooping easier, and Desiree was then able to scoop 4 bites without help, and needed only a little help from her mother to scoop 5 more bites. Recommendation also made for use of rubber mat (such as shelf liner) under bowl to keep it in place, and grandmother reports she will bring some from her house. Improved ability to feed herself with a spoon shows good progress toward expected outcome of Desiree feeding herself all meals without help. Plan to address drinking from sippy cup next session as mother has stated goal to "get her off the bottle."

DEPARTMENT OF HEALTH AND HUMAN SERVICES
CENTERS FOR MEDICARE & MEDICAID SERVICES

PLAN OF TREATMENT FOR OUTPATIENT REHABILITATION
(COMPLETE FOR INITIAL CLAIMS ONLY)

1. PATIENT'S LAST NAME	FIRST NAME Emma	M.I. S.	2. PROVIDER NO. XXXXXX	3. HICN XXXXXX
4. PROVIDER NAME Jennifer S , OTR/L	5. MEDICAL RECORD NO. *(Optional)* XXXXXX		6. ONSET DATE 4/13/11	7. SOC. DATE 5/5/11

8. TYPE ☐ PT ☒ OT ☐ SLP ☐ CR ☐ RT ☐ PS ☐ SN ☐ SW	9. PRIMARY DIAGNOSIS *(Pertinent Medical D.X.)* Parkinson's (332.0); pneumonia (482.9)	10. TREATMENT DIAGNOSIS Malaise & fatigue 780.79	11. VISITS FROM SOC.

12. PLAN OF TREATMENT FUNCTIONAL GOALS	PLAN
GOALS *(Short Term)* 2 wks: Client will demonstrate: 1. Bed mobility with min assist & adaptations to use bedside commode. 2. SBA with sit↔stand transfers to bed and toilet using walker. 3. Ability to complete grooming activities in standing with SBA. 3 wks: Client will demonstrate: 1. Dressing with min assist. 2. Bathing with min assist OUTCOME *(Long Term)* 6 weeks: In order to perform ADLs at home, client will demonstrate: 1. Independence in mobility & transfers for ADLs/IADLs. 2. Independence in toileting using commode or bathroom. 3. Independence in w/c mobility. 4. Independence in dressing and bathing.	• ADL retraining • Transfer & functional mobility training • Adaptive equipment training • Safety education • Client / Caregiver Education • Therapeutic exercises for strengthening • Neuromuscular re-education for balance

13. SIGNATURE *(professional establishing POC including prof. designation)* Jennifer S , OTR/L	14. FREQ/DURATION *(e.g., 3/Wk. x 4 Wk.)* 3/wk X 6 wks

I CERTIFY THE NEED FOR THESE SERVICES FURNISHED UNDER THIS PLAN OF TREATMENT AND WHILE UNDER MY CARE ☐ N/A	17. CERTIFICATION
15. PHYSICIAN SIGNATURE	16. DATE	FROM 5/5/11 THROUGH 6/4/11 N/A

18. ON FILE *(Print/type physician's name)*
☐

20. INITIAL ASSESSMENT *(History, medical complications, level of function at start of care. Reason for referral.)*	19. PRIOR HOSPITALIZATION
	FROM 4/13/11 TO 4/16/11 N/A

Client is a 73y.o. female who lived alone and did accounting work until hospitalized for pneumonia 4/13/11. She is temporarily residing at her daughter's home where she received 2 wks of home health OT. Client was referred to outpatient OT by Dr. Cole on 5/3/11. Client states she wants to return home and return to prior level of independence in self care, transfers, mobility, and IADLs, including tax preparation. Medical hx and complications include Parkinson's Disease and several falls. Cognition: Alert and oriented X 3. ADL tasks: Mod assist in bathing and dressing due to fatigue from illness and complications of inactivity and Parkinson's Disease. Client feeds self after set-up. Mobility: Client needs mod A for bed mobility, min A for transfers, and CGA for ambulation with wheeled walker for safety. Client is propelled in w/c by her daughter due to fatigue, balance, and ambulation difficulties. AROM is WFL but client is slow to initiate movements. Strength is 4/5 in bilateral UEs. Grip strength is 10# on right, 8# on left. Client is motivated and rehab potential is excellent for return town home with possible homemaker services or Meals-on-Wheels assistance. Client would benefit from skilled OT instruction in safe use of adaptive devices, self-care and IADL, transfer techniques, and home evaluation.

21. FUNCTIONAL LEVEL *(End of billing period)* PROGRESS REPORT   ☐ CONTINUE SERVICES **OR**   ☐ DC SERVICES

22. SERVICE DATES
FROM   THROUGH

Form CMS-700-(11-91)

Figure 14-1. Centers for Medicare & Medicaid Services Form CMS-700.

DEPARTMENT OF HEALTH AND HUMAN SERVICES
CENTERS FOR MEDICARE & MEDICAID SERVICES

UPDATED PLAN OF PROGRESS FOR OUTPATIENT REHABILITATION
(Complete for Interim to Discharge Claims. Photocopy of CMS-700 or 701 is required.)

1. PATIENT'S LAST NAME	FIRST NAME	M.I.	2. PROVIDER NO.	3. HICN
	Emma	S.	XXXXXX	XXXXXX

4. PROVIDER NAME	5. MEDICAL RECORD NO. *(Optional)*	6. ONSET DATE	7. SOC. DATE
Jennifer S , OTR/L	XXXXXX	4/13/11	5/5/11

8. TYPE	9. PRIMARY DIAGNOSIS *(Pertinent Medical D.X.)*	10. TREATMENT DIAGNOSIS	11. VISITS FROM SOC.
☐ PT ☒ OT ☐ SLP ☐ CR	Parkinson's (332.0); pneumonia (482.9)	Malaise & fatigue (780.79)	11
☐ RT ☐ PS ☐ SN ☐ SW	12. FREQ/DURATION *(e.g., 3/Wk. x 4 Wk.)* 3/wk X 4 weeks		

13. CURRENT PLAN UPDATE, FUNCTIONAL GOALS *(Specify changes to goals and plan.)*

GOALS *(Short Term)* 2 wks: Client will: 1. Perform sit↔stand transfers to bed, toilet, and commode independently. 2. Manage clothing during dressing, bathing and toileting CGA for balance after set-up. 3. Demonstrate safe transfers and mobility with SBA from caregiver during home evaluation.

OUTCOME *(Long Term)* 4 wks: In order to perform ADLs in her own home, client will demonstrate 1. Independence in bed mobility & transfers. 2. Independence in toileting, dressing, bathing after set-up. 3. Safe and independent use of walker and w/c during ADLs in home.

PLAN
- ADL retraining
- Transfer & functional mobility training
- Adaptive equipment training
- Safety education
- Client / caregiver education
- Home evaluation

I HAVE REVIEWED THIS PLAN OF TREATMENT AND RECERTIFY A CONTINUING NEED FOR SERVICES ☐ N/A ☐ DC	14. RECERTIFICATION FROM 6/5/11 THROUGH 7/4/11 N/A
15. PHYSICIAN SIGNATURE	16. DATE	18. ON FILE *(Print/type physician's name)* ☐

18. REASON(S) FOR CONTINUING TREATMENT THIS BILLING PERIOD *(Clarify goals and necessity for continued skilled care.)*

Client has made significant progress in 4 wks as demonstrated in her ability to complete supine to sit with CGA using a bed rail and a firmer mattress. Client needs SBA with sit↔stand transfers to/from bed; ambulates with wheeled walker SBA for safety to/from bathroom. Client now able to propel self in w/c independently from bedroom to kitchen and bathroom but requires daughter's assistance to propel w/c outdoors. Demonstrates good awareness of safety precautions by using brakes during transfers. Client progressed from mod assist to min assist in dressing and bathing but requires help managing clothing, doing fasteners, and bathing back when standing due to ↓ balance and AROM. Client would benefit from continued ADL retraining, transfer and mobility training using assistive devices, skilled instruction and a home evaluation of mobility and safety issues during ADLs at home with caregiver assistance. Rehab potential is excellent for discharge to her own apartment in 4 wks.

19. SIGNATURE *(or name of professional, including prof. designation)* Jennifer S , OTR/L	20. DATE 6/5/11	21. ☐ CONTINUE SERVICES OR ☐ DC SERVICES

22. FUNCTIONAL LEVEL *(At end of billing period – Relate you documentation to functional outcomes and list problems still present.)*

	22. SERVICE DATES FROM THROUGH

Form CMS-701(11-91)

Figure 14-2. Centers for Medicare & Medicaid Services Form CMS-701.

Consultation

Consulting work is another area of occupational therapy practice that may use a slightly different method or language for documentation. Occupational therapists may consult on a wide variety of questions about which they have special expertise. For example, a psychiatric unit that relies on recreational therapists and activity aides for its activity therapy program might ask for an OT consult on a client who has both physical and psychiatric disabilities. A newborn nursery might ask for an occupational therapy consult on a high-risk infant. An occupational therapist may be asked to evaluate a work, home, or school setting to make recommendations regarding safety, adaptations for work simplification, ergonomics, energy conservation, or compliance with ADA standards. An OT consultant might be used to peer review charts for quality improvement monitoring or for reimbursement issues.

A consultant gives a professional assessment of what needs to be done, rather than actually doing it. Two of the most common requests for occupational therapy consultations are for consultation on individual consumers, or for consultation on the context in which the consumer works or resides.

Individual Consumers

A consult on an individual consumer is written in the consumer's health record, just as any OT note would be. In a problem-oriented medical record, the note is written in chronological order in the progress note section in a SOAP format. In a source-oriented record, the consult would more likely be written in a different format, and would be found in the section of the record marked "consults." It might be in the form of a letter or memo, or it might be written on some kind of form that the consulting OT uses routinely. The following note documents a consultation provided for a psychiatric client who had positioning needs, and is written in SOAP format so that you can see how that would be done. In Chapter 15, there is an example of a consultation on an individual client done in a different format.

Occupational Therapy Consult
Date: 9/12/11   Time: 10:30 AM   Positioning Consultation
Mr. E was seen at the request of Dr. Andrews to evaluate his positioning needs.

S: *Consumer reports that he is not able to find a comfortable position in his wheelchair, and that he is not able to propel it in a straight line due to a drag on one of the wheels.*

O: *Consumer noted to be leaning to the Ⓡ with increased pressure on the Ⓡ elbow. Back of wheelchair noted to be hammocking badly. Arm rests do not provide a good position for functional use of arms. Gel cushion in chair seems to be working well as an anti-pressure device but transfers cold to consumer. Upon inspection, wheel found to have hairs wound around the axle, and also in need of oiling.*

A: *Several changes in the wheelchair are needed to increase comfort and functional use:*
- *Add an anti-sling insert to the back of the chair to provide a more upright posture.*
- *Add a pad to the gel cushion to prevent cold transfer of gel to consumer and also for ease of cleaning in case of incontinence.*
- *Ⓑ arm bolsters are needed for w/c arm rests to bring consumer's arms closer to midline for ↑ functional use.*
- *Clean and oil wheels at axle.*

P: *The adaptations listed above have been ordered. Consumer to be re-evaluated after the wheelchair is repaired and adapted.*
Lisa P, OTR/L

Settings in Which the Consumer Works or Resides

In evaluating a client's home or workplace prior to discharge, a SOAP note might also be used. For an example of a home evaluation, see Chapter 15. However, if a work setting were evaluated for ergonomic correctness or for ADA compliance as a whole rather than in relation to one specific client, a letter or standardized evaluation form would be more appropriate. The following letter documents a work site evaluation that was done on a consulting basis.

MEMO
To: Earl Y, R.Ph.
From: Charlet Q, OTR/L
Re: Computer ergonomics in the pharmacy
Date: April 14, 2011

On the above date, a visit was made to the 2nd floor pharmacy in response to your request to perform an ergonomic evaluation of the computer work stations located there. This is in response to complaints of carpal tunnel pain and neck and shoulder discomfort. The following are my recommendations:

1. *Computer keyboards must be positioned low enough so that the shoulders can be relaxed during sustained usage and so that wrists can be maintained in neutral position rather than in extension or flexion. When the wrist is in extension or flexion, there is more stress on the median nerve that is compressed in the carpal tunnel and may cause pain.*

   The best position may be achieved by lowering some of the keyboards and/or angling them so the wrists can be kept neutral. Sometimes keeping the keyboards flat or even inclining them with the far end slightly down may help keep the wrists in neutral position. A wrist rest used in conjunction with the keyboard is helpful to some users.

   If an ergonomic keyboard is used to avoid wrist deviations, it still must be positioned so the wrists are not either flexed or extended. The correct position for each person will be slightly different since all body builds are different. It will be important for each user to know the correct body mechanics and be able to make some adjustments in the workstation to meet his/her needs.

2. *The chair should support the back well while maintaining the trunk in an upright position (not leaning back or forward). Thighs should be supported and the entire foot should be supported while sitting in a chair at a computer station. Foot support may be either the floor or a footrest (flat or angled) as needed to support the feet. The rungs attached to the high stools do not allow adequate foot support and may tend to disrupt back alignment. Adjustable-height chairs are recommended to meet individual needs.*

3. *The monitor needs to be placed directly in front of the viewer so it is not necessary to maintain a rotated position of the neck and trunk. Several monitors were angled to the side, requiring the user to maintain asymmetrical posture, causing neck and back strain. The height of the monitor should be adjusted so the eyes of the viewer look directly forward onto the upper one-third of the screen. This prevents neck strain, which can occur if the viewer is having to look up for sustained periods of time.*

4. *If the mouse is to be used with any frequency, it should be positioned near the keyboard rather than requiring a forward reach. A wrist rest attached to the mouse pad is preferred to remove stress from the heel of the hand.*

5. *Ideally, it seems that the computer workstations should be lowered from high counters to normal table or desk work-height. Table-top should ideally be 26" from floor and the distance eye to screen should be 26" to 30". However, it is possible to manage the existing problems with the correct chairs, footrests, monitor positioning, and keyboard/mouse positioning.*

6. *Taking a break every 30 minutes to do some active movement and stretching exercises is recommended. A copy of sample exercises was left in the pharmacy.*

If you plan to purchase chairs, footrests, etc., it would be best to actually go to an office supply vendor to try out specific pieces of furniture, or arrange to have the items on loan so the potential users can check the fit. I hope this is helpful. Please let me know if I can be of further assistance.

Charlet Q, OTR/L

DOCUMENTATION IN PALLIATIVE CARE

Occupational therapists who work in hospice settings or in other practice settings where clients have terminal illnesses often provide palliative care rather than rehabilitation. Palliative care provides comfort, relief from symptoms, and quality of life as clients prepare for death. In this situation, there is no expectation that the client will make progress in physical functioning. Goals often center around pain control, energy conservation, maintaining independence in areas of occupation that are meaningful to the client, obtaining adaptive equipment, and family/caregiver education. Relaxation, active listening, and complementary and alternative therapies are often used with hospice clients. The note below shows one of the complementary/alternative therapies (Tai Chi) being used to increase relaxation and social participation and to maintain activity tolerance, balance, functional mobility, and satisfaction with quality of life.

Jean is a 48-year-old woman whose throat cancer was diagnosed late and has now metastasized to the brain. She is a single woman who has devoted her life to her career in one of the health professions. She understands her prognosis and has entered a home-based hospice program where she receives occupational therapy as a part of her care. Jean wants to maintain her social participation and her independence in basic and instrumental ADL activities as long as possible. She has always been physically active, but many of the physical activities she has enjoyed doing with friends are too strenuous for her limited energy.

S: *Client states "I feel so much better after doing Tai Chi with you guys, even on days when I think I'm too tired or just don't feel like I'm able to do anything."*

O: *Client participated in 45-minute session in her home with 2 friends present to increase social participation, decrease risk of falling, and incorporate energy conservation techniques taught last week into everyday tasks. Five minutes of warm-up exercises focused on breath-awareness and relaxation were followed by 15 minutes of modified therapeutic Tai Chi with one 5-minute rest period. Client touched chair back as needed for stability during movements requiring weight shift and balance on one foot. Gentle push hands activity was used to challenge balance and to provide physical contact and social engagement during movement activities. Friends remained for short visit and refreshments on the deck, and plans were made to repeat the activity as tolerated in 1 week. Home instruction sheets and a Tai Chi video with relaxation music were provided for use as desired over the next week.*

A: *Client's home bound status, decreased balance, and variable energy levels limit her social participation and IADL activities. Her perception of increased energy and activity tolerance following the Tai Chi activity allows her to continue to engage in occupation she values. Using furniture as props allows client to practice weight shifting and balance in a safe environment. Physical contact and social exchange during push hands reduced social isolation and distress of "not being able to do anything." Client would benefit from continued Tai Chi activities to address energy conservation, balance, and safety concerns through breathing and relaxation activities done in a social setting.*

P: *Client to be seen in her home weekly for 45 minutes or as tolerated for 3 more weeks for instruction in mobility, balance, energy conservation techniques to maintain functional mobility, IADL tasks, and valued role as a friend in a modified home exercise energy conservation program.*

Sandy M, PhD, OTR/L

DIFFERENT FORMATS FOR NOTES

Remember that SOAP is just a format—an organizational structure that may be used for any type of note. An initial evaluation can be written in a SOAP format, as can a treatment or progress note. There are other styles of notes that may be used instead.

Checklists, **flow sheets**, and other similar forms created by the facility are often used instead of SOAP notes to save time. Forms are an especially popular way to document an initial assessment because they allow quite a lot of information to be communicated with little time spent writing. The evaluation/re-evaluation/discharge form presented in Chapter 13 was developed by Capital Region Medical Center in Jefferson City, Missouri (see Figure 13-1). It is a particularly good example because it covers a lot of areas in a small space without sacrificing the ability to individualize the information. It also documents the areas of occupation before the underlying factors so that no time is wasted documenting underlying factors that do not impact function. Using the same form for evaluation, re-evaluation, and discharge allows the reader to evaluate progress toward goals easily. There is ample space for comments so that the form can easily be individualized.

Narrative notes are not formally organized into sections the way SOAP notes are. Narrative notes may present any information in any order desired. Good narrative notes usually contain the "A" data of the SOAP note. Narrative notes reporting primarily the "A" data are becoming more popular due to time and space constraints.

DAP notes are an adaptation of the SOAP format used in some facilities. In this format, the "D" (data) section contains both the "S" and the "O" information.

BIRP, PIRP, or **SIRP notes** are sometimes used in mental health practice settings. Information in this format is distributed as follows:

B: The behavior exhibited by the client

I: The treatment intervention provided by the therapist

R: The client's response to the intervention provided

P: The therapist's plan for continued treatment, based on the client's response

P: The problem/purpose of the treatment

IRP for intervention, response, and plan, as stated previously

S: The situation

IRP for intervention, response, and plan, as stated previously

If you work in a facility that uses one of these formats, you categorize your information slightly differently than you do when you are writing a SOAP note.

ELECTRONIC DOCUMENTATION

In the past several years, electronic health records (EHRs) have become the norm rather than the exception, and they are used in numerous health care settings (Carter, 2008). There are packages available to schedule our days as well as to send and receive mail, to compile our occupational profiles and intervention plans, to write our notes, and to remind us when everything is due. Software packages for electronic systems offer us a menu from which to choose the initial evaluations we want to use and for recording the data. Other packages offer us choices of problems, goals, objectives, and possible intervention strategies rather than requiring us to compose these for individual clients. Such software can make our job simpler and save valuable health care dollars. However, there are some critical issues to be aware of when using electronic documentation systems (Weir & Nebeker, 2007).

First, there is so much information available in an EHR that it is often difficult to locate the particular piece of information or form that you are looking for. Rather than being able to scan quickly through the sections of a paper health record, EHRs may require a user to click through multiple lists and menus to locate the desired item.

Second, it is tempting to copy and paste information from one record to another if the clients have similar issues. This can result in problems ranging from small errors (saying "her" instead of "his") to major errors in accuracy regarding the client's status. Best practice is to enter the information for each client without use of a copy and paste method.

EHRs have also reduced the amount of face-to-face and phone communication between members of the health care team. While electronic documentation is a time saver, you should always remember the importance of collaborating directly with other members of the client's health care team to optimize the quality of your OT services and to maximize your client's outcomes.

Perhaps the most important issue when using EHRs is to remember the importance of developing a rapport with your client and including him or her throughout the OT process.

There is a temptation to interact solely with the computer in selecting goals, objectives, and treatment strategies, particularly if you are using a computer in the treatment room. This practice should be avoided, regardless of the extra time involved in setting goals and choosing intervention strategies **with** the client rather than **for** the client. Effective treatment requires the teamwork of the client and therapist working toward mutually selected and agreed-upon goals.

Finally, there needs to be a way to individualize each section of the treatment plan or note. A good program will allow editing options or places for comments so that the documentation can be individualized to the client. One way to make an effective compromise between selecting from a menu and individualizing the statements is to use a "mix-and-match" system in which the menu offers components of the statement and allows the therapist to choose the components appropriate to the individual client. For example, in Chapter 12 we looked at critical care pathways for clients who have many of the same needs, and earlier in this chapter we examined mix-and-match treatment intervention plans in mental health. In some situations, it is also possible to standardize contact or progress notes. In summary, we need to make certain that the client is our main focus, fitting the software to the client needs rather than fitting the client into the capabilities of the software package.

In the note below, the computer supplies the words in bold, and the therapist completes the sentences:

S: *When asked, client able to state 3/4 hip precautions correctly.*

O: *Pt. participated in 30 minute OT session bedside for skilled instruction in following hip precautions during personal ADL tasks.*

ADLs: Client able to dress upper body ① and lower body modified ① using adaptive equipment with 2 verbal cues to remember hip precautions.

Functional Mobility: Client supine → sit ①, able to walk to bathroom using wheel walker c̄ verbal cues to avoid external rotation when turning.

Contributing Factors: Strength/endurance: Client able to lift 4 pounds using Ⓑ UEs. Rest break needed after 5 minutes of light activity.

Home Program:

A: ***ADLs***: *Ability to remember 3 out of 4 hip precautions when asked and to incorporate 2 of the 4 successfully into his ADL routine shows good progress and good potential to follow hip precautions after discharge.*

Functional Mobility: *Need for verbal cues to follow hip precautions during bathroom tasks results in continued safety concerns.*

Contributing Factors: *Overall deconditioning has resulted in weakness and lack of activity tolerance needed to complete ADL routine without several rest breaks. Client continues to make steady gains in strength and activity tolerance and has good potential to meet goal of ① in ADL tasks after discharge.*

Client would benefit from *continued instruction in incorporating hip precautions into daily activities and from a schedule that increases activity tolerance and overall conditioning.*

P: ***Client to be seen*** *twice daily for 1 more day to complete skilled instruction using adaptive equipment for dressing; to teach tub, shower, and car transfers; and to instruct caregiver in home program.*

Megan M, OTR/L

This program cues the therapist to remember areas that need to be covered in the note and provides the words that must be repeated in every note. There is still opportunity for maximum flexibility in individualizing the documentation. You will note that she did not fill in the blank for home program since she has not yet taught that program. She could omit that section when printing her note, or she could put "Not yet taught."

Figure 14-3 shows an example of electronic documentation that allows the OT to document the initial evaluation, the plan of care, and the discharge summary all in the same report. You will see that this form includes several tables for entering data common to a work hardening setting as well as the option to include a standardized description of the tests that were performed. You will also note some abbreviations not covered in this manual that are specific to the work hardening setting:

+ PRE: Progressive resistive exercise
+ CV: Coefficients of variance
+ PILE: Progressive isoinertial lifting evaluation
+ PDC: Physical demand characteristics

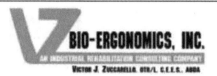

WORK HARDENING EVALUATION – SUMMARY REPORT
Initial Evaluation Date: 4/1/10
Exit Evaluation Date: 4/28/10

Name	Chet D.	
Age	40	
Height (inches) - **72**	**Weight** (lbs) - **250**	**Dominance** (L/R handed) – **R**
Physician: Dr. Lance Sawbones	Follow-up Physician Appointment: 4/30/10	
Diagnosis	s/p L4-5 Fusion	
Date of Injury	1/2/10	
Mechanism of Injury/Medical Tx (as reported by patient)	"Lifted a box at work and felt a pull in my back". Conservative tx for 2 weeks including PT, medications, and time off w/o relief. MRI (+) for large HNP. Fusion 2/1/10 & PT 2/22 to 3/15/10. Attempted return to work on 3/18/10 but unable to tolerate. Rx for Work Hardening written 3/25/10.	
Employer & Job Title	XYZ Corporation – Order Filler	
Insurance Carrier/Adjuster	Coverall Insurance/Sue Payer	
Case Manager	Nancy Nurse, RN, CCM	

Work Hardening Program Attendance:

Attended 18/18 visits for up to 7 hour days. No tardies.

Work Hardening Treatment Program:

Aerobic exercise, stretching/stabilization, PRE, functional tasks, and body mechanics education.

Work Hardening Exit Evaluation Performance Criteria Profile:

Consistency of Effort – CVs low. Cross validation in PILE v. Occasional lifts acceptable.
Quality of Effort – HR during evaluation >/= 25% variance. Acceptable kinesiophysical signs.
Non-Organic Signs – Subjective reports consistent with test behavior. Complaints specific.

Work Hardening Exit Evaluation Assessment:

Significant progress noted in program. He is currently meeting all return to work goals. See the work requirements/goals v. demonstrated physical tolerances on the following page. Feasibility for success at return to work is **GOOD** at this time.

Work Hardening Exit Evaluation Recommendation/Plan:

Pending physician f/u and exam, I recommend return to work at full duty at this time.

Chet D.   Page 1

Figure 14-3. (Reprinted with permission of Vic Zuccarello, OTR/L, C.E.A.S. II, ABDA Owner - BIO-ERGONOMICS, INC.) (continued)

Vic Zuccarello, OTR/L, C.E.A.S. II, ABDA

Work Hardening Evaluation	Chet D.	Page Two

Demonstrated Physical Tolerances

Task	Initial Eval – 4/1/10	Exit Eval – 4/28/10	Job Description	Met? (yes/no)
Pain Level (0-10)	6/10	**3/10**	*Job Description Information (Goals to be Met)Provided By: Employer & Employee*	
Chief Complaints	Midline lumbar aching into R hip.	**Midline lumbar aching.**		
Material Handling Lifting in pounds unless stated otherwise/Push/Pull in Pounds of Force (Occ. = 0-33% of day, Freq. = 34-66%, Const. = > 66%) or (Occ. = 1-12/hr, Freq. = 13-60/hr, Const. = > 60/hr)				
Floor to Waist Lift	25# occasional	**75# occasional, 35# frequent**	**70# occasional, 25# frequent**	**MET**
Waist to Shoulder Lift	"	"	"	**MET**
Overhead Lift	"	**50# occasional, 25# frequent**	**40# occasional, 20# frequent**	**MET**
Carrying (50 feet)	"	**75# occasional, 35# frequent**	**70# occasional, 25# frequent**	**MET**
Pushing (Force)	55#	**100#**	**Pallet jack, dolly**	**MET**
Pulling (Force)	43#	**97#**	"	**MET**
Non-Material Handling Positions and movements in activities and associated tasks (Occ. = 0-33% of day, Freq. = 34-66%, Const. = > 66%) or (Occ. = 1-12/hr, Freq. = 13-60/hr, Const. = > 60/hr)				
Standing	Occasional	**Frequent**	**Frequent**	**MET**
Walking	"	"	"	**MET**
Squatting/Bending	"	"	"	**MET**
Kneeling/Crawling	"	**Occasional**	**Occasional**	**MET**
Reaching/Grasping	Frequent	**Constant**	**Constant**	**MET**
PDC Level (S,L,M,H,VH)	**MEDIUM**	**HEAVY**	**HEAVY**	**MET**
Perceived Disability	Oswestry – 44%	**Oswestry – 22%**		

Physical Demand Levels of Work *Dictionary of Occupational Titles (US Dept. of Labor, Fourth Edition, Revised 1991)*

PDC Level	Occasional (0-33% of day)	Frequent (34-66% of day)	Constant (>66% of day)
Sedentary	*1# to 10# /* Stand & Walk	*Negligible/* Sitting	*Negligible/* Sitting
Light	*11# to 20#*	*Up to 10# /* Stand & Walk *and/or* Standing pushing/pulling controls	*Negligible and/or* Seated & pushing/pulling arm/leg controls
Medium	*21# to 50#*	*11# to 25#*	*Up to 10#*
Heavy	*51# to 100#*	*26# to 50#*	*11# to 20#*
V-Heavy	*Over 100#*	*Over 50#*	*Over 20#*

END OF SUMMARY

Chet D.   Page 2

Figure 14-3 (continued). (Reprinted with permission of Vic Zuccarello, OTR/L, C.E.A.S. II, ABDA Owner - BIO-ERGONOMICS, INC.) (continued)

Example of Work Hardening Evaluation Data Pages (from Chet's Initial Evaluation)

LUMBAR MUSCULOSKELETAL SCREEN

Resting HR	84 (min acceptable increase = 105)		Resting BP	124/66
Pre Pain Level	5/10		Description	Midline lumbar and R hip
Posture	increased lumbar lordosis, protruding abdomen, PSIS even, no shift.			
Gait	mild R antalgia		Palpation	increased muscle density lumbar PVM's

NEUROLOGICAL

	L	R	Comments
Knee Reflex (L4)	2+	2+	symmetrical
Ankle Reflex (S1)	"	"	"

WADDELL SIGNS
(+) = abnormal response to examination, or possible non-organic sign

TENDERNESS		SIMULATION		DISTRACTION		REGIONAL		OVER-REACTION
Superficial	-	Axial loading	-	L SLR +	R SLR -	Cogwheel	-	-
Non-anatomic	-	Simulated rotation	-	Sit 75	Sit 75	Numb	-	
				Supine 30	Supine 55	Weak	-	

RANGE OF MOTION
(Pre test AROM take 3 trials and calculate coefficient of variance; CV >15% = Inconsistent Test)

MOTION	PRE TEST (°)			AVERAGE (°)	CV%	POST TEST (°)	NORM
Lumbar flexion	35	30	35	33	7.1	30	60
Lumbar extension	10	10	12	11	8.8	15	25
L lateral flexion	20	22	22	21	4.4	15	25
R lateral flexion	20	25	25	23	10.1	25	25

STATIC STRENGTH

MOTION	TRIALS			AVERAGE	CV%	Manual Muscle Test
R knee flexion	34.4	36	40.1	36.8	6.5	4
L knee flexion	26	25	22	24.3	7.0	5
R knee extension	77.3	88	80.2	81.8	5.5	4
L knee extension	33	31	25	29.7	11.5	5
R plantarflexion	33.3	30	34	32.4	5.4	4
L plantarflexion	36.2	36	32	34.7	5.6	5
R dorsiflexion	22	24.4	18.6	21.7	11.0	4
L dorsiflexion	20	22.6	20.6	21.1	5.3	5

QUALITY OF MOVEMENT (Non-Material Handling) SCREEN (5x each)

Squatting	full, UE assist required	Overhead Reach	full, fluid, unguarded
Bending	50%	Finger Flexion	as above
Kneeling	full, UE assist	Opposition	as above
Crawling	symmetrical, guarded	Climbing	step to step, decreased RLE WB.
Comments	Guarding in lower level postures.		
Post-Pain Level (0-10)	6/10 – no change in location of symptoms. Denies need for break, "let's go".		

Chet D.   Page 3

Figure 14-3 (continued). (Reprinted with permission of Vic Zuccarello, OTR/L, C.E.A.S. II, ABDA Owner - BIO-ERGONOMICS, INC.) (continued)

Work Hardening Evaluation	Chet D.	Page Four

Material Handling Test

Description of lift/carry test: This test format is based on other commercial lifting tests and utilizes a lifting box and weights. The worker is instructed in proper body mechanics, the therapist demonstrates proper procedure, and the worker is then allowed to perform a preferred number of practice trials. After each successful lift, weight is added in progressive fashion and the worker is asked if the load is "light, medium, or heavy". The worker is also asked if they feel safe to perform the lift with heavier weight. If the worker answers with a "yes" response and the form on the previous load was safe, weight is added (5-10# for a 'heavy' response, 10-15# for a 'medium' response, and 15-20# for a 'light' response) until one of three termination criteria are met: physiological (ie heart rate, perspiration, flushed complexion); kinesiophysical (ie recruitment of surrounding body parts, substitution, counterbalancing, muscle tremor)); or psychophysical (ie desire to stop because of 'heaviness' of load, perceived pain, or perceived cardiopulmonary exertion). During the test, these aspects of performance are observed and utilized to determine if the worker provided acceptable effort, and if the worker's subjective reports are in proportion with test behavior. Maximum safe effort is solicited and encouraged. The worker is never forced to perform a task they feel is unsafe.

- 50-foot Carrying is assessed by first testing with the max load achieved in the waist to shoulder lift and progressing as in the above procedure.
- Upon reaching the end-point, the load is decreased by 50% and 10 repetitions are performed to determine the frequent carrying load.

Description of push/pull test: Static testing is performed to assess for level of participation in testing as well as to elicit a measure of pushing/pulling strength. The worker is instructed in safe technique (including by not limited to avoidance of jerking or holding the breath, etc.), the therapist demonstrates proper procedure, and a preferred number of practice trials are performed. The worker then performs 6-second trails at their own preferred safe-maximum force. A maximum rest period of 15 seconds is given between 3 trials. Therapist observes for physiological (heart rate, flushed complexion, perspiration); kinesiophysical (substitution, recruitment, tremor, counterbalancing); and psychophysical (pain level, heart rate v. rate of perceived exertion) indicators. Maximum safe effort is solicited/encouraged, but subject is not coerced into providing higher force than they feel is safe.

Pre-test Heart Rate	**90**	**Pre-test Pain Level**	**5/10**

Test	Load (#)	Heart Rate	Rate of Perceived Exertion (6-20)	Pain Level (0-10+)	Kinesiophysical Indicators
Floor to waist lift	25	114	14-15/20	6	Counterbalance and recruitment
Waist to shoulder	25	114	13-14/20	6	"
Overhead Lift		110	14-15/20	6	"
* Carrying Max	25	110	15-16/20	6	"
Pushing (force)	55	115	11-12/20	6	"
Pulling (force)	43	122	"	6	"
Comments:	Body mechanics were safe and steady. HR and kinesiophysical signs suggest acceptable effort.				

END OF EVALUATION

Chet D.   Page 4

Figure 14-3 (continued). (Reprinted with permission of Vic Zuccarello, OTR/L, C.E.A.S. II, ABDA Owner - BIO-ERGONOMICS, INC.)

Chapter 15

Examples of Different Kinds of Notes

This chapter provides examples of notes from a variety of stages of treatment and from a variety of practice settings. The first group of notes illustrates different stages of treatment and the second set provides examples of single treatment sessions in different practice settings.

CHAPTER CONTENTS

EXAMPLES OF NOTES FOR DIFFERENT STAGES OF TREATMENT

EXAMPLES OF NOTES FOR DIFFERENT PRACTICE SETTINGS

Gateley CA, Borcherding S. *Documentation Manual for Occupational Therapy: Writing SOAP Notes, 3rd Edition* (pp. 189-210)
© 2012 SLACK Incorporated

The notes in this chapter were written by students, faculty, and practicing therapists. The signatures are chosen to make the notes anonymous. Required demographic information is not included on all notes due to space considerations.

INITIAL EVALUATION REPORT: HIP FRACTURE

Name: Rebecca B   *Age*: 80   *1° Dx*: Ⓛ *hip fx*   *2° Dx*: *HTN*
Funding Source: Medicare
Admission Date: 5/02/11   *Date of Referral*: 5/03/11
Estimated Length of Stay: 4 days   *Physician*: Dr. Garrett

Brief Occupational Profile: Ms. B reports living alone and being Ⓘ in all ADLs prior to admission. She had gone upstairs to use the bathroom since there was none on the first floor. She became light-headed, fell down the stairs, and broke her hip. She was admitted for a total hip replacement yesterday. Her family lives out of town and cannot stay with her. She wants to return home. Ms. B has supportive neighbors and lives in a small town where she is retired from her position as a second grade teacher. She lives across the street from the elementary school and is in the habit of visiting with the children and some of their families when school is out each day. She is also active in her church.

Occupational Therapy Note
Date: 5/03/11   *Time*: 8:30 AM
S: Client stated that she would like to "get this leg well" and go home to "live a regular life."
O: Client participated in 45-minute ADL eval in room to assess capabilities following Ⓛ THR. Client educated on use of ADL equipment for self-care tasks and adherence to hip precautions. Client demonstrated ability to repeat 2/4 precautions. During ADL evaluation, client was observed flexing 8° to 10° beyond 90° and required 4 verbal cues to remain at or below 90° during the 45-minute session. Other 3 hip precautions were followed. Client able to complete sponge bath at sink p̄ set-up for upper body, and used dressing stick with washcloth and verbal cues for lower body. Client partial wt. bearing on Ⓛ leg; required min Ⓐ for balance with sit ↔ stand to bathe back peri area. Client able to complete upper body dressing after set-up. Client able to don underwear and pants over hips using a dressing stick with min Ⓐ. Client able to don socks using sock aid with min Ⓐ. Client able to complete grooming tasks and oral care Ⓘ from w/c level. Following verbal cues, client demonstrated good problem solving by trying different body positions to perform ADLs while adhering to hip precautions and demonstrated understanding of adaptive aids by utilizing reacher and dressing stick correctly after instruction. Client demonstrated ↓ activity tolerance as she required four 2-minute rest breaks during dressing tasks. Client then taken to OT clinic for evaluation of client factors:

Ⓑ UE AROM: WFL   Ⓑ UE strength: WFL
UE sensation: Intact   Grip strength: Ⓡ 47#, Ⓛ 43# (Ⓡ-hand dominant)
Tripod pinch: Ⓡ 10#, Ⓛ 5#   Lateral pinch: Ⓡ 10#; Ⓛ 5#

A: Client's motivation, problem-solving skills, and understanding of equipment use indicate excellent rehab potential. Upper body strength and AROM WFL are beneficial to learning adaptive techniques for self-care and functional mobility. ↓ endurance, ↓ balance, and inconsistent compliance with hip precautions present safety concerns during lower body dressing and bathing. These problem areas negatively impact client's ability to be safe and Ⓘ with ADLs. Client would benefit from skilled instruction on hip precautions and use of adaptive equipment with ADL performance, therapeutic activities which facilitate dynamic standing balance, and ↑ ADL activity tolerance. Exploration of interim living arrangement or possible continued home visits and home equipment procurement will be needed if progress warrants discharge to home.
P: Client to be seen b.i.d. for 1 hour the next 3 days to ↑ Ⓘ in self-care tasks through instruction on hip precautions and use of adaptive equipment, with tasks to ↑ activity tolerance, and dynamic standing activities.
LTG: By anticipated discharge on 5/07/11 client will:
   ❖ Safely complete lower body dressing and bathing modified Ⓘ utilizing adaptive equipment with 100% adherence to hip precautions.
   ❖ Safely complete toileting mod Ⓘ using adaptive equipment (walker & bedside commode).

STG:

   ❖ *By next tx. session, client will complete toileting with SBA for sit ↔ stand from bedside commode and manage clothing with no more than 2 verbal cues.*
   ❖ *By 2nd session, client will don shoes & socks 100% of time with modified Ⓘ, utilizing adapted techniques & devices with 100% adherence to hip precautions.*
   ❖ *By 3rd session, client will complete all lower body dressing tasks with SBA using adaptive equipment with no more than one 30-second rest break.*
   ❖ *By 3rd session, client will complete toileting with SBA using wheeled walker and commode frame over toilet.*
   ❖ *By 4th session, client will safely bathe her peri area modified Ⓘ utilizing adaptive techniques and devices with 100% adherence to hip precautions.*

Kim N, OTR/L

INTERVENTION PLAN: HIP FRACTURE

Name: *Rebecca B*   **Age**: *80*   **1° Dx**: *Ⓛ hip fx*   **2° Dx**: *HTN*
Strengths: *UE strength & AROM WFL; intact cognition and motivation to return home*

Functional Problem Statement #1: *↑ fatigue, ↓ endurance for ADLs, and inconsistent compliance with hip precautions makes client unsafe in ADL tasks.*
LTG #1: *By anticipated discharge on 5/07/11, client will safely complete lower body dressing and bathing modified Ⓘ utilizing adaptive equipment with 100% adherence to hip precautions.*

STG (Objective)	Interventions
STG #1: *By 2nd session, client will don shoes & socks 100% of time with modified Ⓘ, using adapted techniques & devices with 100% adherence to hip precautions.*	1. *Instruct & have client verbalize 4/4 hip precautions.* 2. *Provide written handout of hip precautions.* 3. *Instruct in use of adaptive techniques/devices followed by demonstration of use in dressing activities.*
STG #2: *By 3rd session, client will complete all lower body dressing tasks with SBA using adaptive equipment with no more than one 30-second rest break.*	1. *Continue instruction in use of adaptive techniques/devices followed by demonstration of use in dressing activities.* 2. *Educate client and provide written instructions on energy conservation techniques. Evaluate understanding by her application during ADL task; ask about how she performs ADL tasks at home.*
STG #3: *By 4th session, client will safely bathe her peri area modified Ⓘ using adaptive techniques and devices with 100% adherence to hip precautions.*	1. *Instruct in use of adaptive techniques/devices followed by demonstration of use in bathing activities.* 2. *Instruct in manipulation of clothing and bathing items while standing in walker at sink s̄ violating hip precautions.* 3. *Assess for home equipment needs and continued home services if progress warrants discharge to home.*

Functional Problem Statement #2: *↓ dynamic standing balance makes client unsafe during ADL tasks.*
LTG #2: *By anticipated discharge on 5/07/11, client will safely complete toileting mod Ⓘ using adaptive equipment (walker & bedside commode).*

STG (Objective)	Interventions
STG #1: *By next tx. session, client will complete toileting with SBA for sit ↔ stand from bedside commode and manage clothing with no more than 2 verbal cues.*	1. *Instruct client in safe transfer techniques; reinforce compliance with total hip precautions.* 2. *Provide UE strengthening through reaching and wt. bearing activities at sink and closet for grooming and dressing items and pushing up from chair and bedside commode.*

STG #2: *By 3rd session, client will complete toileting with SBA using wheeled walker and commode frame over toilet.*	1. *Continue instruction in safe transfer techniques; reinforce compliance with total hip precautions.* 2. *Interview client regarding home environment; explore and discuss interim living arrangements or possible equipment use & placement in home; discuss support services needed if discharge home is warranted.*

INITIAL EVALUATION: SEATING AND MOBILITY

Seating and Mobility Evaluation
Name: *Kaycie B*   **DOB**: *4/03/1994*   **Date of Eval**: *7/07/11*   **Age**: *17*
Primary Dx: *Incomplete C6 SCI due to MVA 5/14/11*   **Secondary Dx**: *Depression*
Funding Source: *Private Insurance Company*

Medical History & Occupational Profile: *Kaycie is a 17-year-old young woman with a diagnosis of incomplete C6 SCI resulting from a motor vehicle accident (MVA) on her prom night. Her boyfriend was killed in the MVA, and Kaycie continues to deal with depression related to that event and her residual functional deficits. Kaycie had no significant medical history prior to the MVA. She will be a senior in high school this fall and enjoys photography and playing piano. She lives at home with her parents and 15-year-old brother. Kaycie has undergone 6 weeks of intensive inpatient rehabilitation. She is being evaluated for a power wheelchair in preparation for discharge home. Kaycie, her mother, and the rehab facility OT attended this evaluation.*

Current Seating/Mobility: *For the last two weeks of her rehabilitation stay, Kaycie has utilized a loaner tilt-in-space power wheelchair on a trial basis. Per client, family, & staff report, Kaycie has been independent with mobility in her hospital room and throughout the facility.*

Home Environment: *(based on report from rehab facility OT) Home is a large one-level ranch with an open floor plan. Family has already made considerable modification to the home including installation of ramp to enter front door, widening of doorways, and renovation of bathroom for w/c accessibility. Kaycie completed a home visit with the facility OT on 7/06/11 and reportedly was able to access the bedroom, living room, kitchen, dining room, bathroom, and patio using the power w/c. Mother reports that an anonymous member from their church has donated a van with a w/c lift.*

Cognitive/Visual Status: *Rehab OT, speech therapist, and neuropsychologist report Kaycie's cognitive and visual perceptual function as WNL.*

ADL Status: *Kaycie is able to complete upper body dressing and bathing with set-up. She requires moderate assistance with lower body dressing and bathing using adaptive equipment. She currently requires maximum assistance for bowel program and catheter management, although rehab team is addressing client and caregiver training this week to increase Kaycie's independence with these tasks.*

UE function: *Kaycie has 4/5 strength throughout her dominant Ⓡ UE. She has 3+/5 strength in her Ⓛ UE shoulder and elbow, and no active movement in her Ⓛ wrist or hand.*

Sensation: *Sensation intact Ⓡ UE; absent in distal Ⓛ UE. Impaired Ⓡ trunk & LE; absent Ⓛ trunk & LE.*

Transfers/Mobility: *Kaycie requires minimal assist for bed mobility with a rail, including supine → sit. Kaycie completes a squat pivot transfer w/c ↔ bed/toilet with moderate assist. She is independent in maneuvering a power wheelchair using a standard joystick. She is also able to operate the tilt-in-space option independently for pressure relief.*

Assessment: *Kaycie is non-ambulatory due to motor impairments resulting from incomplete C6 SCI. She is unable to propel a manual w/c independently due to significant impairments of Ⓛ UE AROM and strength as well as decreased strength in Ⓡ UE. Kaycie is not a candidate for a scooter as she would not be able to transfer safely into a scooter seating system or operate the tiller driving system effectively. Therefore, the use of a power wheelchair is necessary to improve Kaycie's ability to participate in mobility-related activities of daily living. Tilt-in-space and air cushion are necessary as Kaycie sits in the w/c for 10+ hours daily and is therefore at high risk for development of pressure ulcers. Kaycie is unable to perform a functional weight shift and unable to transfer independently to the bed for pressure relief.*

Without this device, Kaycie would be at risk for decreased ability to participate in mobility-related activities of daily living such as accessing the bathroom for bathing and toileting and accessing the dining room for family meals. She would have no independent, safe, or effective means of mobility or function within her home, school, or community. Additionally, she would be at significant risk for development of pressure sores, postural deformity, and pain.

Recommendation: Recommend purchase of the following to accommodate Kaycie's body dimensions, postural alignment, and pressure relief needs:

- 18" X 16" power wheelchair with power tilt-in-space
- Push-button lap belt
- Desk-length flip-up height-adjustable armrests with standard joystick mounted on right armrest
- Removable headrest
- Rear anti-tippers for stability during tilt of wheelchair
- Ankle straps & heel loops to maintain feet on footplates
- Air cushion with incontinence cover to prevent pressure ulcers
- Lap board for UE support during feeding and school activities
- Standard tires & casters with flat free inserts.

Plan: Kaycie will discharge home using existing loaner wheelchair from this company. Upon insurance approval of the above recommendations, equipment will be delivered to Kaycie's home for fitting and training in safe and effective use. Follow-up appointments will be conducted as needed for modification of equipment.

Francesca M, OTR/L, ATP, RTS

INTERVENTION PLAN: CANCER

Name: Carol M   *Age*: 35   *Primary Dx*: Mastectomy $2°$ breast CA

Strengths: Prior to surgery, Carol was in good physical condition and employed full-time. She has some social support from her sister who lives in another state.

Functional Problem Statement: Carol avoids social outings with friends due to ↓ self-esteem secondary to cosmetic alterations imposed by mastectomy procedure, which precludes her ability to return to work.

Long-Term Goal: Carol will ↑ social interactions and activity to 6 outings/month within the next month, in preparation for return to work.

STG (Objective)	Interventions
STG #1: Carol will identify one support group of interest to her within 1 week in order to ↑ willingness to be out in public for work and social activities.	1. Educate Carol re: available support groups and peer visitation groups, their contact persons, and their telephone numbers, and ask her whether she has made contact. 2. Ask if Carol would like to have her contact information given to a volunteer from the hospital's peer mentor group.
STG #2: Carol will attend 1 support group activity within 2 weeks in order to ↑ confidence in social and work situations.	1. E-mail and/or phone call to remind Carol of upcoming support group meetings. 2. Discuss with Carol her experiences with the support groups.
STG #3: Carol will initiate conversation with at least one other support group member during her first visit to the group in order to ↓ negative impact of cosmetic alterations to body image.	1. Accompany Carol into the community the first time she goes out. 2. Encourage participation in group discussion.
STG #4: Carol will enroll in a women's exercise program in order to ↑ activity tolerance and positive body image.	1. Educate Carol re: area exercise groups for post-mastectomy clients. 2. Follow-up phone call to ask if she has enrolled in an exercise program.
STG #5: Carol will identify 5 assets she possesses other than physical in order to ↑ self-esteem and confidence in social and work situations.	1. Discuss Carol's assets with her, encouraging her to think of as many as she can. 2. Educate Carol regarding books and Web sites that address post-mastectomy concerns.

Functional Problem Statement: Carol is unable to return to work 2° 3/4 AROM, 4-/5 muscle strength, ↓ activity tolerance (fatigues after 1 hr.), and sensory changes.

Long-Term Goal: Carol will return to work part-time by 8/08/11.

STG (Objective)	Interventions
STG #1: Within 2 weeks, Carol will complete 2 hours of work tasks with no more than one 15-minute rest break.	1. Scar massage and myofascial release to incision area along with client education on self-massage. 2. PROM to Ⓛ shoulder—instruct in self-ranging program. 3. Work simulation tasks.
STG #2: Carol Ⓘ will retrieve 5 items from overhead shelf using Ⓛ UE in work simulation task within 3 weeks.	1. Active resistive ROM to Ⓛ UE. 2. Resistive strengthening with thera-tubing, weights, and graded functional activities. 3. Work simulation tasks.
STG #3: Within 3 weeks, Carol will transfer twenty 5# boxes from one table to another in <10 minutes using Ⓑ UEs with reported pain level <2/10.	1. Work simulation with client education on energy conservation principles. 2. Provide home exercise program and modify as client progresses.
STG #4: Within 3 weeks, Carol Ⓘ will use correct body mechanics in seated and active work tasks in order to have pain level of <2/10 while working.	1. Educate in ergonomics and posture in order to prevent pain. 2. Provide education on women's exercise groups.
STG #5: Carol Ⓘ will demonstrate sensory precautions in work and daily living tasks within 2 weeks.	1. Provide education on safety concerns with sensory loss. 2. IADL tasks and work simulation with sensory hazards to check application of safety techniques.

RE-EVALUATION: WORK HARDENING (FACILITY FORMAT)

Note: This example contains abbreviations specific to a work hardening setting that are not listed in Chapter 4.

Work Hardening Re-evaluation
Worker: Joe Fireman   **Date**: 7/07/11   **DOB**: 2/29/79   **Age**: 33
Employer: Gotham City   **Job Title**: Firefighter/Paramedic
Physician: Dr. Pain   **Dx**: s/p Ⓛ shoulder reconstruction   **Attendance**: 5/5 sessions

Subjective Data
Subjective Complaints: Pain level was rated as 3-4/10 pre-test and post-test. He described sharp pain near the left acromioclavicular (AC) joint, with aching in the anterior/posterior deltoid and into the left upper trapezius musculature.
Work Plan: Return to his usual and customary job when able.
Perceived Disability: Worker scored 14/70 on the Pain Disability Index, which indicates a low level of self-perceived disability. This represents a moderate improvement from 39/70 upon initial evaluation.

Musculoskeletal Screen
Musculoskeletal Deficit Changes Since Last Eval: In comparison to the unaffected right shoulder, slight ROM gains are noted with the Ⓛ UE, while still remaining below expected AMA norms. Left shoulder strength is 5/5 within the given range (exception for external rotation 4+/5), while Ⓡ UE strength is 5/5 in all planes. Occasional sustained forward/overhead reaching task continues to be completed at an above competitive proficiency level
Quality of Movement Changes: Functional overhead reaching and internal/external rotation with the Ⓛ UE has improved, but remains decreased vs Ⓡ UE. Mild decreased control was noted with the Ⓛ UE with maximum load handling at all levels. Mild compensation patterns were observed with use of Ⓛ UE when crawling and climbing ladders.

Summary of Demonstrated Abilities

Material Handling	Max. Occasional (lbs.)			Employer-Reported Job Requirements
	Entrance (5/03/11)	Re-Eval (5/17/11)	Re-Eval (6/07/11)	
Floor - Waist Lift	55	60	70	May lift >100 lbs from floor to chest or shoulder height in emergency scenarios (occas.); may handle tools up to 45 lbs floor to overhead (up to frequent as needed)
Waist - Shoulder Lift	20	45	55	
Shoulder - Overhead Lift	15	35	40	
Bilateral Carry	60	60	70	
Unilateral Lift/Carry (L/R)	30/55	55/55	55/55	
Pushing (force) (L/R)	73 (31/42)	57 (31/31)	89 (39/51)	Up to 70# (hands in front); up to 35# overhead push/pull with pike pole
Pulling (force) (L/R)	70 (33/37)	57 (35/25)	80 (41/39)	
Non-Material Handling	**Frequency Displayed**			**Job Requirements**
Sitting	Unrestricted	Unrestricted	Unrestricted	Occasional
Standing	Unrestricted	Unrestricted	Unrestricted	Frequent
Walking	Unrestricted	Unrestricted	Unrestricted	Frequent
Climbing	Limited	Improved	Frequent	Frequent
Bending	Unrestricted	Unrestricted	Unrestricted	Frequent
Reaching (Forward/ Overhead)	Occasional/ Limited	Occasional/ Limited	Frequent	Frequent
Squatting/Kneeling	Unrestricted	Unrestricted	Unrestricted	Frequent
Crawling	Occasional	Occasional	Up to Frequent	Occasional

Consistency and Quality of Effort

Client continues to provide good and consistent effort with testing, based upon positive HR response to activity, low coefficients of variation (CV) values with ROM/static strength tests, and the presence of external effort indicators. Please see chart below for description of criteria.

Global Effort Rating: Consistency and Quality of Effort Indicators

Criterion	Result	Comments
Pain Diagram: Reports of circumferential pain, glove or stocking presentation would in most cases be supported in the literature as inconsistent with the diagnosis.	Expected	No unusual markings for given diagnosis.
Pain Behavior and Function: High pain ratings should be consistent with altered movement patterns and range of motion. Alteration of movement patterns should be consistent in associated tasks/transitional movement patterns v. direct measurement. A patient's behavior should consistently reflect distress, and not only during performance of evaluation tasks.	Expected	Pain level was rated as 3-4/10 pre-test, up to 5/10 with testing, and as 3-4/10 post-test. Subjective reports were consistent with displayed function.
Perceived Disability Score: In the absence of organic findings, high-perceived disability may compromise recovery from injury.	Expected	Client's score on the Perceived Disability Inventory (14/70) indicates a low level of self-perceived disability at this time.
Coefficients of Variation: Repeated test trials must be low to indicate consistent effort.	Expected	Worker displayed high CV values during 0 of 10 ROM tests and 0 of 6 static strength tests.
5-Position Grip (bell-curve): Deviation from bell-curves may indicate sub-maximal effort, especially when performed on non-hand diagnoses.	Expected	Worker displayed modified bell-shaped distribution on right/left.

Cross-Reference Validity Check: *Tests repeated at intervals with full volitional effort with >20% variation may be indicator of sub-maximal effort.*	*Expected*	*Variance between results for position 2 on standard grip test and Maximum Modified Voluntary Effort (MMVE) test was 12.1-18.8%.*
Static Force Curve Analysis: *Force curves during static trials should follow a predictable pattern. Delayed and/or erratic force curves may indicate that maximal effort was not achieved during that test.*	*Expected*	*During static strength testing, delayed peak contractions and erratic force curves were noted during 0 of 18 trials.*
HR and RPE Correlation: *A patient's report of physical exertion (RPE) should correlate with a corresponding increase in working heart rate.*	*Expected*	*Working HR and corresponding RPE values were proportionate in all instances.*

Impression

- Client has provided high levels of effort while attending 5 scheduled sessions on the most recent prescription, resulting in additional gains with heavy load handling, pushing/pulling ability, and tolerance for sustained work simulated activities. He continues to wear his turn-out gear during sessions to simulate completing essential job functions.
- Mr. Fireman has displayed safe function in at least the Medium work demand level, with some function into the Heavy demand level, up to the above-listed tolerances. The abilities displayed with testing this date do not meet the employer-reported essential job demands. The main factors limiting return to work continue to be decreased tolerance for the required work demand level, decreased load handling ability, decreased push/pull tolerances, decreased tolerance for sustained work tasks involving the Ⓛ UE (reaching, tool use), decreased active ROM for overhead job tasks, and his subjective pain complaints at this time.

Plan

Mr. Fireman has a follow-up appointment with physician 7/08/11. We will await your recommendations.
Shelia T, OTR/L, CEAS

RE-EVALUATION NOTE: DRIVER REHABILITATION

Driving Re-evaluation

Name: *Charles C*   **Age**: *71*   **Dx**: *Multiple TIAs*

S: Client reports successful completion of 6-week Mature Driver Improvement Course recommended during initial evaluation 2 months ago. "I do okay during the day, but I'm afraid to drive at night. I just don't see that well." Client declined opportunity to drive on 4-lane highway during on-road assessment, indicating that he only drives short distances in his small community and relies on family for longer distance transportation.

O: Client participated in driving re-evaluation this date to determine safety and independence with community mobility. Previous evaluation 2 months ago revealed minor hearing deficits, decreased reaction times, mild left inattention, and impaired ability to recognize and understand road signs.

In-Clinic Evaluation: Visual acuity WFL with bifocal lenses; depth perception WFL. No left inattention observed. Client scored WFL on brake reaction time test. Client correctly identified meaning of 29 of 30 road signs (missed side road intersection sign).

On-Road Evaluation: Client completed 20 minutes driving in car in residential and commercial areas of a suburban area. Results are as follow:

- Client demonstrated proper use of mirrors and over-the-shoulder checks; observed and responded to turn signals of other drivers by slowing down and obeyed all road signs and traffic control devices. Client demonstrated adequate visual scanning when entering the roadway and at all intersections.
- Client correctly used turn signals at appropriate times and activated horn, headlights, and emergency flashers when instructed to do so.
- Client observed posted speed limits and made appropriate adjustments to speed related to intersections, traffic flow, and roadway surfaces. Client demonstrated proper vehicle positioning while moving forward in traffic and before, during, and after all turns.
- Client demonstrated appropriate time and space judgment when changing lanes and negotiating intersections. Client demonstrated adequate brake, accelerator, and steering control when driving forward, backing up, merging, and parking.

A: *Improvements noted in visual perception, reaction time, cognition (understanding road signs), and functional driving performance as compared to initial evaluation 2 months ago. Client's performance this date indicates ability to operate a motor vehicle safely in residential and commercial environments. Decreased night vision and comfort level with driving on busy highways pose safety concerns for driving in those situations. Client would benefit from continued family assistance for night-time or long-distance transportation.*

P: *It is recommended that client's driving be restricted to daylight hours in rural and small town areas. Client should not drive at night or on large, busy highways. Recommendations have been discussed with client and family. They voice understanding that the results of this evaluation are indicative only of the client's functional driving ability on this date. Any changes in health or cognition that would impact driving should be addressed through follow-up with client's physician for potential referral to a Certified Driving Rehabilitation Specialist (CDRS).*

Jeffrey S, OTR/L, CDRS

Adapted from content in *Documenting Driver Rehabilitation Services and Outcomes,* Shipp & Havard, 2006.

PROGRESS NOTE: HAND THERAPY CLINIC

Occupational Therapy Progress Note
Date: 6/07/11   **Time**: 1:00 PM

S: *Client reports pain @ the ulnar styloid with forearm supination. Client reports she is still unable to start her car c̄ her Ⓡ hand but can now use it to turn a doorknob.*

O: *Client participated in 30-minute hand clinic visit for functional range of motion in UE. Moist heat applied to Ⓡ hand and forearm for 10 minutes prior to beginning treatment.*
A/PROM measurements for Ⓡ hand and forearm are:
Key: [Flexion/extension; ( ) PROM; -extension lag; +hyperextension]

Ⓡ *hand*	*MP*	*PIP*	*DIP*
Index	*0/90*	*0/105*	*0/75*
Long	*0/90*	*0/105*	*0/80*
Ring	*0/90*	*0/105*	*0/80*
Small	*0/90*	*-14/105 (0/105)*	*0/79*

Ⓡ wrist: +45/40 composite (+60/50) composite +45/50 noncomposite
Ⓡ forearm: supination 62 (78); pronation 90
Client performed the following exercises c̄ Ⓡ UE: Isometric forearm supination x10, AAROM supination x5, AROM forearm supination x5. After exercise, client's supination ↑ to 77° AROM. HEP revised to include blue foam for flexion strengthening 2 to 3x day.

A: *Client's gains in DIP flexion AROM since last week is due to ↑ strength of flexors. Active wrist extension ↑ 9° and extension ↑ 5° from last week. ↑ in active pronation is due to ↑ strength while client lost 14° of forearm supination since last week, which appears to be a result of muscle tightness. Client would benefit from continued skilled OT to regain functional ROM to complete IADLs and for general strengthening.*

P: *Client to be seen 2x/wk. for 30-minute sessions. Continue wrist exercises and modify treatment plan to include more supination stretching and strengthening.*

Laurie D, OTR/L

PROGRESS NOTE: INPATIENT MENTAL HEALTH

Occupational Therapy Note
Date: 5/19/11   **Time**: 1600

S: *During the first 2 days of admission, Ms. J elected not to attend OT group sessions, maintaining that she was too "anxious and overwhelmed."*

O: *Client stayed in her room most of the time for first 2 days despite consistent invitations to attend groups. On this day, the client attended a stress management group. Initially she was quiet, but gradually began entering into the activity. She was able to identify specific physical, emotional, and behavioral symptoms that she experiences when feeling overwhelmed or anxious. Ms. J stated that she previously had not been aware of these stress reactions.*

A: *The client is making progress as indicated by her initiating attendance to group, as well as relaxing and opening up socially during the group. Additional progress indicated by recognizing specific symptoms of stress as opposed to relating only general feelings. Client would benefit from participation in daily OT groups focused on stress management.*

P: *Continue all goals as originally stated. Client to be seen daily for 3 days to provide opportunities for Ms. J to learn basic stress management techniques so that she may recognize and control stress reactions when she begins feeling overwhelmed or anxious.*

David L, OTR/L

Progress Note: Community Mental Health

Transitional Housing Facility Monthly Progress Note

Name: *Marco*   **Date**: *November 30, 2011*

1° Dx: *Schizophrenia*   **2° Dx**: *Substance abuse*

S: *Client reports feeling "very stressed" thinking about the upcoming holidays and "having to do what my family wants me to do. They think just because I have schizophrenia, I'm also stupid." Client also reports feeling "great" about his ability to maintain sobriety for 1 month.*

O: *Client completed first month at transitional housing facility. OT attendance, participation, and goals addressed are summarized below:*

Group Participation

Group Name	# Attended	Full Participation
Cooking Club	2 of 3	2
Procovery	2 of 4	2
House Meeting	4 of 4	4
Health Class	4 of 4	3
Substance Abuse	2 of 3	2
Grocery Shopping	3 of 4	3
Leisure Trips	3 of 4	3

Individual Service Participation

1-on-1 Appointments	#
Completed	7
No Shows	0
Cancelled/Rescheduled	0
1-on-1 Hours	**#**
Total Spent with OT	6 hrs
Total Spent with OTS	2 hrs

Goals Addressed During Groups & Individualized Service Meetings

	Access/Linkage/ Transportation	X	Computer Skills		Hygiene/Self-care		Medical Health	X	Self-Esteem
X	Advocacy (Personal/political)	X	Cooking		IADL Assessment	X	Mental Illness Education	X	Substance Use
X	Anger/Emotion/ Stress Mgmt		Discharge Planning	X	Interpersonal Skills		Non-grocery Shopping	X	Symptom Mgmt
	BADL Assessment		Education/GED		Laundry/ Clothing Care	X	Nutrition/Meal Planning	X	Time Mgmt
X	Budgeting/Money Handling		Family Support/ Development	X	Leisure/Social		Problem Solving		Vocational/Work
	Bus Training	X	Goal Setting		Literacy	X	Routine/Schedule and Organization		Volunteering/ Productive Occupation
	Cleaning/Home Care	X	Grocery Shopping		Medication Mgmt		Safety		Others (specify below)

Family Interactions: *Client set a plan for self-advocacy with family with max verbal cues. Following interpersonal skills training, client requested to contact family members to practice new skills. In two 30-minute visits, client demonstrated reciprocal conversation without outbursts, accusatory statements, or passive-aggressive behaviors.*

Sobriety: *Despite noted stressors, he was able to independently follow sobriety plan he created at admission.*

Internet Use: *Client able to access novel and routine Web sites of choice with min verbal cues (required mod Ⓐ at admission) required for impulsivity and attention to task.*

IADLs: *Client completed grocery shopping with min verbal cues for item location and price comparison (required mod Ⓐ at admission). Client declined to work on budgeting/savings plan this month due to spending all his income on the upcoming holidays. Client indicated desire to budget next month with intent to save $50 toward a television set for his room.*

A: *Stress related to family perceptions and expectations results in ineffective interactions with family members. Ability to participate in reciprocal conversation without negative interactions demonstrates progress toward goals. Sobriety for 1 month indicates great progress toward client's goal of refraining from drug & alcohol use. Impulsivity and decreased attention to task limit client's independent Internet usage, but decreased need for verbal cues this month indicates progress. Continued need for assistance with budgeting and grocery shopping limit client's ability to transition to more independent living situation, but progress with grocery shopping indicates good potential for this goal. Client would benefit from continued group and individual service participation in this transitional housing facility to address limitations in social interaction, sobriety, Internet usage, and independent living skills.*

P: *Client to attend all scheduled weekly groups and twice-weekly individual OT sessions to address social participation, sobriety, Internet usage, and independent living skills. Plan to help client establish and follow monthly budget, increase social contact with family, maintain sobriety plan, and increase independence with Internet usage.*

Stephanie S, OTR/L, QMHP

PROGRESS NOTE: BALANCE AND VESTIBULAR REHABILITATION

Name: Juanita S   *Age*: 73

1° Dx: Ⓛ *peripheral vestibulopathy*   *2° Dx*: *OA, CAD, Ⓑ cataracts*

S: *Pt. reports continued feelings of spinning, blurred vision, and difficulty walking. She reports she has not completed the home exercises provided two weeks ago because they make her feel dizzy and she gets scared. She also reports needing to hold onto the shower door for support when stepping in/out of the tub. No recent falls reported.*

O: *Client participated in 45-minute balance session in outpatient OT clinic to address balance deficits identified during initial eval. 2 weeks ago.*

Current Status: *Client is able to keep eyes forward on target and perform 10 reps of slow head turns with report of increased dizziness from 1 to 3 (0 = no symptoms, 10 = most extreme symptoms). Client is able to follow visual target up and down with report of dizziness from 1 to 3 (same scale). With min verbal cues, client able to increase speed of head movements without further increase in reported dizziness.*

Client education: *Client was re-educated regarding the balance system, her dx, the reason for OT, and the importance of consistency with her home exercises for balance; client voiced understanding. HEP modified to accommodate client's comfort level with exercises, and she demonstrated ability to complete:*

  ❖ *Steady gaze with head turns*

  ❖ *Following visual target vertically, horizontally, diagonally during IADL task (putting away dishes)*

Pt also instructed to have family member present for safety when bathing; voiced understanding. Written recommendations provided to client and reviewed with daughter at end of session.

A: *Continued report of dizziness and habit of holding onto shower door during shower transfer indicate safety concerns with ADL & IADL tasks. Decline in dizziness rating (3/10) this session shows progress from initial evaluation rating (6/10). With consistent performance of HEP and continued balance & vestibular rehabilitation, client has potential to decrease dizziness and increase her safety in her independent living situation.*

P: *Continue OT 1x/wk for 4 wks to address safety concerns related to symptoms of Ⓛ peripheral vestibulopathy. Sessions to focus on increasing client's tolerance of head movements without increased dizziness and client education regarding compensatory strategies for increased safety during ADLs & IADLs.*

Patricia D, OTR/L

TRANSITION PLAN: REHAB

Date: 2/15/11   *Time*: 09:00 AM

S: Client said "I feel so much better than I did a while back. I feel like I've come a long way."

O: Client participated in 15/20 scheduled tx sessions from SOC, with last few sessions focused on transition planning from inpatient to skilled nursing setting. Client illness prevented attending 5 sessions. OT sessions focused on ADL retraining, toileting, functional transfer training, ↑ AROM, and strength. Client level of function at transition is as follows:

Goals	Initial	Transition
Dressing: UE ① LE ①	Min Ⓐ for balance Mod Ⓐ for balance	Set-up CGA when standing to don underwear & pants
Bathing: UE ① LE ①	Min Ⓐ Min Ⓐ	① Modified ① using long-handled sponge
Transfers: sit ↔ supine ① stand ↔ w/c & toilet ①	SBA Min Ⓐ	SBA SBA
AROM – WFL Ⓑ	Shoulder abd 65° (strength 2) Shoulder flex 55° (strength 2) Elbow 0-125° (strength 3-)	Shoulder abd 90° (strength 3) Shoulder flex 60° (strength 3) Elbow WFL (strength 4)

A: Client exhibited an increase in AROM and strength. Client has met bathing and hygiene goals. Dressing and transfer goals partially met. Client continues to make progress and would benefit from further OT intervention to increase UE strength and activity tolerance to perform ADLs ① and meet all goals.

P: Discharged from inpatient occupational therapy 2° change of status from Medicare Part A → Medicare B. Request physician's orders to re-evaluate under Medicare B in SNF. Upon physician's orders, recommend skilled OT intervention 3x week to increase activity tolerance and strength to perform ADLs ①.

Carrie C, OTR/L

DISCHARGE NOTE: SOAP FORMAT

Client: Ted D   *Admit Date*: 1/29/11
OT Order Received: 2/07/11   *OT Evaluation Completed*: 2/08/11
Number of Treatments: 5   *Discharge Date*: 2/16/11

S: Client reports "doing a lot better" and being "less confused" than he was on admission.

O: Client initially presented with multiple trauma 2° to MVA. OT evaluation on 2/08/11 indicated client had deficits in short-term memory, safety awareness, attention to task, and ADL status. Client participated in 5 OT sessions of ADL retraining for dressing and grooming and functional mobility. Client and family received skilled instruction in safety precautions in the home. Client's functional status on admit and discharge as follows:

Goal #	Admit Status	Goal	Discharge Status
1	Min Ⓐ in grooming	Set-up/supervision	Set-up/supervision
2	CGA toilet transfers	SBA	SBA
3	Supine → sit c̄ min Ⓐ	SBA	SBA
4	Min Ⓐ UE dressing	Set-up/supervision	Set-up/supervision

A: All goals achieved due to improved cognitive status, awareness of safety precautions, and skilled instruction in ADLs. Client will need supervision at home 2° remaining cognitive (attention and short-term memory) deficits.

P: Client discharged to home. Recommend home health OT evaluation for safety in home environment and potential for necessary durable medical equipment. No home exercise program given. No other referrals at time of discharge. OT will follow-up in 1 month by phone to check client's functional status in the home.

Alissa Z, OTR/L

DISCHARGE NOTE: FACILITY FORMAT

Name: Marjorie P   **Health Record #**: 97865
Physician: Dr. Dietrich   **Start of Care**: 4/01/11
Room: # 537   **Date of Discharge**: 4/10/11
Primary Dx: CVA   **Secondary Dx**: Arthritis

_X_ Occupational Therapy   _ Physical Therapy   _ Communicative Disorders

Course of Treatment: Client participated in 30-minute sessions daily for 9 days following CVA to work on ↑ independence in self-care skills, functional mobility, UE strengthening, energy conservation, and activity tolerance.

Status at Discharge: Client reports feeling much better and is ready to go home.

Admit Status	**Discharge Status**
Self-care mod Ⓐ	Self-care Ⓘ and safe
Functional mobility mod Ⓐ	Functional mobility Ⓘ and safe
Activity tolerance 7 minutes for ADLs	Activity tolerance 10 minutes for ADLs

Goals Met: Client has met self-care and functional mobility goals using energy conservation techniques.

Goals Not Met: Activity tolerance goal not met due to client declining last 2 treatment sessions when she learned she was being discharged.

Client/Family Education: Client instructed in and demonstrates understanding of HEP. Handouts provided. Client reports having weights at home she can use for continued UE strengthening as instructed in her HEP.

Recommendations: Discharge client to her sister's home due to goals being met. HEP attached. No home health recommended at this time.

Haley B, OTR/L

CONSULTING NOTE: OUTPATIENT PEDIATRIC CLINIC

This consulting note is not done in a SOAP format since it is designed to be sent to the school rather than written in the child's health record. This note also provides an example of a note that is done by a student co-signed by the supervising occupational therapist.

Hospital and Rehabilitation Center - Motor Skills Clinic
Name: Brianne Elyse Sample   **Date of Birth**: May 20, 2006
Date of Evaluation: July 25, 2011   **Chronological Age**: 5 years, 2 months
Parents: Russ and Jamie Sample
Phone: (555) 888-3988

Brianne Elyse Sample is a 5-year, 2-month-old girl who is being seen today upon request of her family and the UMC Kindergarten Program. Brianne was an active, healthy child until April of 2011, at which time she developed Haemophilus influenzae type-B meningitis. Brianne was hospitalized for 10 days and had a "long recovery" by the family's report. Even though Mr. and Mrs. Sample feel that Brianne has now made a full recovery, they are concerned that this illness slowed her previously fast progress and that she may not be ready for kindergarten this fall. The parents and the UMC Kindergarten Program are requesting an evaluation to assess her readiness for kindergarten.

Assessment Results: Three subtests of the Peabody Developmental Motor Scales, 2nd edition (PDMS-2, 2000) were administered to Brianne on July 25, 2005. The PDMS-2 is a standardized norm-referenced evaluation designed to assess fine and gross motor skills in children birth to 71 months of age. Today's evaluation of Brianne (at chronological age 5 years, 2 months) reveals:

Subtest	*Standard Score	Percentile Rank	Age Equivalent
Object Manipulation	11	63rd	5 years, 11 months
Grasping	10	50th	5 years, 3 months
Visual-Motor Integration	11	63rd	5 years, 8 months

*Standard scores are based on a mean of 10 and a standard deviation of 3.

Brianne's combined performance on the grasping and visual motor integration subtests resulted in a Fine Motor Quotient (FMQ) of 103 (mean of 100, standard deviation of 15), placing her in the 58th percentile for overall fine motor skills.

Brianne was alert and cooperative throughout the 25-minute evaluation. She exhibited a right hand dominance, utilizing the right upper extremity as the main initiator of activity and the left upper extremity as an assist and stabilizer. Posture, muscle tone, strength, and endurance all appeared to be within normal limits for chronological age. Response to auditory stimuli in the environment was appropriate. The parents do not report any hearing or vision concerns. During the evaluation, the child did not squint, rub eyes, nor exhibit any difficulties with visual regard/tracking.

Summary: *Results of the three subtests of the PDMS-2 (given on July 25, 2011) indicate that Brianne Elyse Sample is functioning slightly above the mean in the area of fine motor skills at chronological age 5 years 2 months. Motor coordination and response to environmental stimuli appear to be within normal limits for chronological age. Even though Brianne was recently hospitalized with a serious illness, she currently exhibits adequate fine motor abilities to perform kindergarten activities.*

Actions Taken: *Evaluation results were discussed with Brianne's parents who attended the evaluation session today. A copy of this report will be sent to the family and to the UMC Kindergarten Program as requested by the family.*

Plan: *Re-evaluation upon request.*

Truman T, OTS   7-25-11   Christy N, PhD, OTR/L   7-25-11

CONSULTING NOTE: ASSISTIVE TECHNOLOGY (FACILITY FORMAT)

Occupational therapists are often members of an assistive technology team when assessing clients for augmentative and alternative communication (AAC) devices or other assistive technology equipment. The following note was co-written by an OT and a speech-language pathologist (SLP). It is not in SOAP format because it is being sent to a local agency for funding of recommended equipment.

Name: *Caitlin R*   ***Age***: *13*   ***Dx***: *Muscular dystrophy*   ***Funding***: *County Agency*

Caitlin participated in consultative appointment at assistive technology clinic to determine effective hardware & software adaptations for independence in computer use.

Subjective: *Caitlin states "I want to be able to use the computer for school stuff, e-mail, and Facebook without my mother helping me." Mother reports that client currently navigates the Internet by telling her mother what to click.*

Hearing: *WNL*

Vision: *Caitlin presented with decreased visual acuity but demonstrated compensation using high contrast, enlarged computer screen, and a large high-contrast cursor.*

Speech & Language: *The client's receptive skills were commensurate with her expressive language skills. She was able to process and follow complex verbal directions for her age. Due to decreased air volume, speaking becomes fatiguing after just a few minutes of conversation.*

Mobility: *Caitlin is independent with mobility using a power wheelchair with mini proportional joystick in a familiar spacious environment.*

Neuromuscular Skills: *Caitlin presents with progressive quadriparesis throughout her body. Due to the nature of her diagnosis, she fatigues very quickly.*

Visual Skills: *The client presents with good visual scanning skills to scan keys on a keyboard and good visual tracking to follow a cursor.*

Sensory Processing: *Caitlin demonstrates good cause/effect understanding and functional attention to access a computer. She demonstrates high motivation to access a computer and the Internet.*

Results of Assistive Technology Assessment: *Caitlin is physically unable to use a standard keyboard or mouse but likes to navigate the Internet by telling her mother what to click. Caitlin was unable to use a joystick mouse, trackball mouse, or glide point. She demonstrated good use of a mini proportional joystick to drive her wheelchair. She does not have Bluetooth capabilities in the electronics of her wheelchair. After observing her use with the mini proportional joystick, Caitlin was presented with an ABC Joystick and an XYZ Mini-joystick, ABC and XYZ onscreen keyboards, USB switch interface, and an ultralight switch. Caitlin demonstrated the ability to move the highly sensitive ABC Joystick and spell on both onscreen keyboards, but preferred the letter contrast and simplicity of XYZ keyboard using small movements of her right index finger and thumb. She clicked on choices using her left hand and the ultralight switch. She was highly successful with this combination and independent to navigate the Internet and spell out* *messages using a word processing document. She also demonstrated the ability to check her e-mail and social networking accounts with the above-mentioned adapted computer equipment. She was unable to move as accurately or quickly with the XYZ Minijoystick. Caitlin also presents with low vision related to the above diagnosis. It was felt during the evaluation that Caitlin would benefit from Text Enlargement Software, which would provide screen reading as well as magnification as needed.*

Recommendations*: As a result of the assistive technology evaluation, it has been determined that Caitlin is an excellent candidate for adaptive software/hardware to allow her improved access to her computer and Internet. It is recommended that she receive an ABC Joystick USB, a USB switch interface, XYZ Keyboard, Text Enlargement Software, and an ultralight switch to increase her independence on the computer and Internet. It is also recommended that Caitlin receive an updated computer system in order to increase her independence with written communication needs.*

Shawna D, MLS, OTR/L, ATP   Michelle W, MS, CCC-SLP

CONTACT NOTE: ACUTE CARE

Occupational Therapy Contact Note
Date*: 4/22/11   ****Time****: 15:00*

S: *Client nonverbal. Client demonstrated startle response c̄ position change.*

O: *Client participated in bedside OT session to work on initiating and attending to self-care task. When asked to point finger, client required multiple verbal cues and demonstrations, and demonstrated poor response time. Client requires max Ⓐ supine → sit EOB. Client required multiple verbal cues and hand over hand Ⓐ 75% of the time to initiate holding on to washcloth. Client able to bring washcloth to water with 1 verbal cue but required hand over hand Ⓐ to bring washcloth to face. Client attended to looking at self in mirror for ~1 minute. Client required hand over hand Ⓐ to initiate brushing hair. Shoulder AROM limited due to ↓ tone.*

A: *Overall, client's motor planning, task initiation, and attention during treatment activities continues to be limited. Client would benefit from ranging activities to increase shoulder elevation, as well as further interventions focusing on the skills of initiating and attending to task in order to complete ADL activities.*

P: *Client to continue OT daily for 20-minute sessions until discharge in ~2 weeks to work on self-care activities and the underlying performance skills and client factors necessary to complete tasks Ⓘ.*

Elyce P, OTR/L

CONTACT NOTE: COGNITION

Occupational Therapy Note
Date*: 4/05/11   ****Time****: 10:00 AM*

S: *Veteran reports feeling fine, but says he does not remember the OTR's name that he has been working with.*

O: *Veteran participated in OT session in clinic for cognitive tasks, Ⓡ UE AROM, strengthening, and fine motor coordination. Veteran oriented to person, month, year, and place after prompting. He followed two-step commands after max verbal cues and mod physical assist to complete basic self-care tasks. Veteran was unable to grasp and release items with Ⓡ hand. He required mod physical Ⓐ and verbal cues to complete UE AROM used in table top activities.*

A: *Decreased orientation to surroundings presents safety concerns. ↓ cognitive functioning leads to ↓ attention to completion of tasks, specifically dressing, feeding, and bathing. Veteran would benefit from cognitive skills training and safety instruction. ↓ strength, coordination, and AROM in Ⓡ UE limits his ability to complete ADL activities. He would benefit from instruction in using Ⓡ UE as an assist as well as from activities to ↑ Ⓡ UE strength, AROM, and coordination to perform self-care activities.*

P: *Veteran will be seen daily for 3 weeks for 1 hour to improve cognitive skills, ↑ attention to task and safety awareness, and to ↑ Ⓡ UE strength, AROM, and coordination in order to complete self-care tasks.*

Taylor M, OTR/L

Contact Note: Complementary/Alternative Therapy (Craniosacral)

As occupational therapists and occupational therapy assistants increase their skills in the use of complementary and alternative therapy techniques, questions arise about how to document interventions that may be focused on client factors and that use nontraditional components such as energy work or chakra balancing. Many of these visits are done on a private pay basis, since complementary therapy is often not reimbursable by either public or private insurance. It is best to report objectively on what was said, what was done, what impact the presenting problems have on the client's ability to engage in meaningful occupation, and what the plan is for continued services, just as you would for any service you might provide.

Occupational Therapy Note
Date: 2/05/11   **Time**: 4:30 pm
S: Client reports ↓ in functional mobility and ↑ pain since hip replacement surgery. He has adaptive equipment and is able to state 3/3 hip precautions. He reports gains since last visit as follows:
- He was able to sleep 4/7 nights without medication and sleeps longer without waking.
- Headaches occur less often.

O: Client participated in 1-hour craniosacral session in clinic to decrease pain and increase functional mobility needed for work and both personal and instrumental ADL activities. He arrives using forearm crutches in place of the walker he used last week. On evaluation, the craniosacral rhythm is asymmetrical, as is the body, with the left side cephalad and the head tilting right. The major restrictions identified are in the pelvis, which is treated first with a series of diaphragm holds, and release of the sacrum in supine. With increased symmetry to the pelvis, the Upledger cranial series ending with a long still-point is used to facilitate homeostatic healing activity in the body.

A: Improvement in sleep (decreased need for pain medication and increase in time asleep from 1 to 1½ hours), decrease in headaches, and graduation from walker to forearm crutches all indicate good progress in treatment, as does visual and palpable increase in pelvic symmetry after today's session. Client would benefit from continued work to the pelvis to alleviate cumulative trauma and residual restrictions from recent hip surgery, followed by work to more subtle restrictions that have resulted from a series of previous serious accidents.

P: Client to return in 1 week, at which time reassessment will determine the frequency, duration, and direction of treatment. As soon as pelvic symmetry is improved sufficiently to allow mobility WFL for work and IADL tasks, regional tissue release can be included to increase the mobility of the head and neck, which is contributing to the headaches.

Sharon B, OTR/L, CST

Contact Note: Early Intervention

Neonatal Follow-Up Outpatient Clinic
Name: Peyton D   **Age**: 11 months   **Primary Dx**: r/o developmental delay
Primary Payment Source: Blue Cross   **Secondary Payment Source**: none

Pertinent History: Peyton is an 11-month, 11-day-old male child whose adjusted age is 9 months, 27 days. He was initially discharged from hospital on May 29, 2010 (chronological age 1 month, 2 weeks; adjusted age 2 weeks). Since discharge, Peyton has been seen twice for medical evaluation at the hospital (8/18/2010 & 12/08/2010). He is being seen today for his first OT developmental evaluation as a part of the Outpatient Neonatal Follow-Up Program. His mother is present at the evaluation.

Occupational Therapy Note
Date: 3/25/11   **Time**: 8:30 AM
S: Child is not yet old enough to use language to communicate, but makes sounds ("ba, da, ma," etc.) WFL for overall developmental level.
O: Today's evaluation reveals:
- Atypical patterns of posture and movement (persistent primitive reflexes, presence of tonic reflexes, moderate increase in muscle tone, limited repertoire of movement, and postural asymmetry).

* Possible visual difficulties (immature visual tracking and intermittent malalignment (one/both eyes drift inward).

* Delayed milestones (child exhibits skills clustering around the 4- to 6-month developmental level).

A: These findings indicate that this child is experiencing developmental delay, deviance in the pattern of development, and possible visual difficulties. Peyton would benefit from the plan of care detailed below.

P: The mother has been informed of the results of the evaluation, and is in agreement with the following plan:

* OT will contact the Neonatal Follow-Up Clinic physician regarding vision concerns.

* Referral made to State Early Intervention program to initiate OT services.

* Peyton scheduled to return to Neonatal Follow-up Clinic on 6/30/2011.

Christy N, PhD, OTR/L

CONTACT NOTE: HOME EVALUATION

Occupational Therapy Home Evaluation Report
Date: 11/08/11   **Time:** 3:40 PM

S: Client stated numerous times how nice it was to be home. Client verbalized more in this setting than at the facility.

O: Prior to admission, client lived at home alone with support from family and home health nurse and housekeeping aide and was Ⓘ with all ADLs. The following are the results of a home evaluation:

Entry: 2 ½" step, 4" door jam. Uneven grass to step. Concrete broken and no railings present.

Kitchen: 26" area around table in center of kitchen, 27" between snack bar and fridge, 30" high snack bar located on outskirt of kitchen. Little room to maneuver safely. Needs utensils and appliances within reach.

Hallway: 22" wide from dining room → bedroom with bathroom between inaccessible for walker. Remainder of entries adequate to accommodate walker.

Bathroom: 17" floor to tub top, 18" floor to toilet seat. Bathroom small, but can accommodate wheeled walker.

Other: Throw rugs in all rooms. Chair blocks bedroom access with wheeled walker. End tables block access to living room from dining room with wheeled walker.

A: With the following modifications and recommendations, the home would be safe for client to return to after discharge:

* Remove all throw rugs to decrease falls; remove excess furniture to increase walking area and increase safety.

* Adaptive equipment needed:

  • Raised toilet seat with safety rails, shower chair with back support, grab bars, and hand-held shower.

  • Add railing to hallway to increase safety without walker.

  • Add railing and repair concrete to outside entry.

* Remove kitchen table and utilize snack bar or dining table to increase mobility in kitchen.

* Lower telephone by back door to improve reach.

P: Resident and family will implement the preceding recommendations and changes to allow discharge from facility to return home safely.

Carrie C, OTR/L

CONTACT NOTE: HOME HEALTH VISIT

Occupational Therapy Note
Date: 2/04/11   **Time:** 8:30 AM

S: Client stated that he was "shaky" from his shower earlier in the AM. Client's daughter reported that client showered and dressed with min Ⓐ for balance and coordination to manage fasteners. Client reported that he has been following his HEP.

O: Client participated in home evaluation to assess balance, coordination, level of compliance, and Ⓘ c̄ HEP and to introduce new hand strengthening exercises. Client required mod verbal cues to initiate and complete pre-existing HEP.

New hand-strengthening exercises added—finger spread with rubber bands of various sizes; intrinsic muscle coordination worksheet (e.g., pen rolling, etc.)

Client and daughter participated in discussion about planning treatment activities to complement client's interests. Gun repair projects and small woodworking activities were suggested for coordination and strength in hands. Client demonstrated good static sitting balance throughout the session, but needed CGA for balance to stand safely from chair.

A: *Need for verbal cues to initiate HEP raises continued concerns about compliance. ↑ strength c̄ Theraband exercises from 1/29/11 indicated through increased repetitions and decreased fatigue. Progress shown by ability to handle 1" items such as pajama buttons, although still has difficulty with smaller items. Rehab potential is excellent. Client would benefit from continued skilled OT to further instruct in energy conservation techniques, safety, and to modify HEP as client continues to progress.*

P: *Client to be seen 2x/wk. for 1 hour sessions to continue work on self-care Ⓘ, with focus on showering and dressing.*

Stacy S, OTR/L

Contact Note: Home Health Mental Health

Name: *John W*   **Date**: *2/14/11*
Beginning Time: *9:00 AM*   **Ending Time**: *10:15 AM*   **LOS**: *75 minutes*
Goals: *2, 4, and 5*

S: *John states that having a bank account instead of keeping all his money in cash in an envelope is very confusing to him, and he is never sure any more how much money he has. He also reported some continuing confusion regarding his medication.*

O: *John participated in home visit to review his grocery needs and for verbal cues to fill his mediset correctly. Skilled instruction provided in meal planning and calculating probable food costs. He was then taken to the bank to withdraw some money, and to a local grocery store to purchase food. At the bank, the teller figured John's account, which confused him. Skilled instruction provided in calculating a bank balance. At the grocery store, John purchased canned fruits and vegetables, ground beef, fresh lettuce, and a loaf of bread. Upon returning home he put the lettuce and meat in the refrigerator independently and consulted his weekly menu planner to determine what he had planned for lunch. John needed 2 verbal cues to fill his mediset with correct doses of all medications.*

A: *Decreased number of cues required to fill mediset correctly indicates progress from 4 cues required last week. Understanding a bank balance is a new skill for John and he needs continued skilled instruction and opportunities to apply his new knowledge before he is able to manage the account independently. He continues to make progress in choosing healthy foods as evidenced by his independent choice of canned fruits and vegetables and the addition of lettuce to his sandwiches. John could benefit from continued skilled instruction in ADL skills such as independent management of medication, food, and money in order to be able to live independently in the community without the support of a professional caregiver.*

P: *John will continue to be seen weekly in his home and community settings in order to work toward independence in meeting his daily needs.*

Alan Thomas, OTR/L

Contact Note: Mental Health (Multiple Groups)

Occupational Therapy Note
Date: *4/14/11*   **Time**: *4:00 pm*

S: *Client reported she is currently not volunteering and has not worked for the past 4 years due to her disability status. Regarding volunteering, she says, "I need the structure," and further stated that she wants to be productive. Currently, client reports she sleeps "too much" and is having relationship problems.*

O: *Client was admitted yesterday and attended 4/4 group sessions today. During expressive therapy group, client participated in baking with the rest of the group, but did not eat anything. When each group member identified current emotions, client identified hers as miserable, angry, very anxious, overstimulated, frustrated, frightened, and alienated. During skills group, client identified a possible problem she may encounter upon discharge to be lack of organization, with her "red-flags" being oversleeping and agitation. Client welcomed suggestions from others restructuring her use of time.*

A: *Client is very perceptive of her emotions and limitations. Her refusal to eat with the group indicates continued appetite disturbance. Client would benefit from information about eating disorders. She would also benefit from* *continued group participation, with emphasis on increasing self-esteem and time management skills. Client's participation in all 4 group sessions today indicates good rehab potential.*

P: *Client will continue to attend all daily group sessions while on the acute unit to work on increasing self-esteem and ability to structure her time.*

Carmen G, OTR/L

CONTACT NOTE: MENTAL HEALTH (ONE GROUP)

The previous note summarized a client's participation in several groups on one day. Some mental health settings, particularly inpatient settings with short lengths of stay, require a note to be written for **each** group that the client attends. The following note illustrates this type of documentation.

Occupational Therapy Note
Name: Jamie D

S: *Client reports unhealthy self-esteem in the form of negative thoughts about herself. She describes feeling "stupid" and "ugly," particularly when she is under stress.*

O: *Client participated in 1-hr self-esteem group in dayroom. Group session was designed to educate participants regarding healthy and unhealthy self-esteem and to instruct on goal setting and other ways to improve self-esteem. Client demonstrated active participation in all group discussion and activities. With encouragement from other group members and facilitator, client set goal for this week to decrease her negative thoughts and to plan for discharge. She independently identified a compensatory strategy to use when she recognizes negative thoughts; her plan is to replace negative thoughts with something more positive such as thinking about how much she enjoys being around her children. Client initiated discussion about setting up appointments for aftercare following discharge.*

A: *Focus on negative thoughts during periods of stress limits client's ability to complete IADL tasks, including caring for her children. Ability to set goals and identify steps to achieving those goals indicates excellent progress this date. Client has great potential to return to independent living. Client would benefit from continued practice in this area and assistance with identifying and replacing negative thoughts.*

P: *Client to attend self-esteem group daily for 3 days to address self-esteem issues that inhibit IADL performance. Sessions to include group discussions, role play, and written discharge plan development, as well as facilitation of setting up aftercare appointments.*

David M, OTR/L

CONTACT NOTE: PEDIATRIC (PRESCHOOL AGE)

Occupational Therapy Note
Date: 9/06/11   *Time*: 3:00 pm

S: *Mary said she wanted to play, but when the task was difficult for her, she said, "You do it. You fix it."*

O: *Mary participated in an OT home visit to work on use of Ⓑ UEs to ↑ spontaneous use of hand as a functional assist, sitting balance while tailor sitting unsupported, and functional mobility, as a prerequisite to self-care and play skills. Mary was engaged during ~90% of the session.*
Bilateral UE Use: Mary required max Ⓐ to pull shirt over stuffed animal's arms with Ⓡ UE while holding it with Ⓛ UE. She spontaneously used Ⓛ hand to assist with stabilizing animal while pulling sleeve over its arm and shoulder c̄ Ⓡ hand. Mary initiated snapping shirt, but needed max Ⓐ to use Ⓛ hand to stabilize shirt while fastening snaps. Ⓑ hands used to hold animal steady during play.
Sitting Balance: Mary required touch cues from stand → sit in walker and mod physical Ⓐ from side sit → cross-legged sit. She demonstrated adequate sitting balance to play for 5 minutes, requiring tactile cues twice to right herself from a lateral tilt.

A: *Improved Ⓑ coordination and increased use of Ⓛ hand as functional assist now ~ 60% of the time indicates progress since last week. Decreased postural control necessitates CGA to maintain upright position when engrossed in an activity. She would benefit from continued skilled OT for activities, which challenge postural support in order to gain protective responses, body righting, and vestibular integration in order to ↑ her Ⓘ during play.*

P: *Mary will be seen weekly for 7 weeks to continue strengthening postural support in order to ↑ her Ⓘ in play activities, promote Ⓑ hand use, and ↑ use of the Ⓛ hand as a functional assist during ADL and play activities.*

Julie S, OTR/L

CONTACT NOTE: PUBLIC SCHOOL

Occupational Therapy Note
Date: 4/12/11

S: *Kylee did not use verbal language to communicate, but did echo words spoken to her.*

O: *Kylee participated in OT session in classroom to work on fine motor skills to prepare for scissors use and improve prehension patterns for writing. After 5 minutes of brushing to decrease tactile sensitivity, Kylee worked on palmar pinch and tripod grasp prehension patterns using a "Fruit Loop" bracelet activity for 20 minutes. Kylee used tongs (in preparation for scissors use) to pull 15 Fruit Loops out of a cup one at a time. Then using a palmar pinch, she placed each Fruit Loop over a pipe cleaner. Five verbal cues were required for task completion.*

A: *Kylee manipulates tongs well and exhibits a good awareness of positioning of tongs within her hands, which is an indicator that proper scissors use will be attained soon. Good attention to task for entire 25 minutes.*

P: *Continue prehension activities 3x/wk. using a variety of media in 20- to 30-minute intervals until proper scissors use goal is achieved.*

Durwood T, OTR/L

CONTACT NOTE: PROSTHETIC ADAPTATION

Name: Daniel P   *Med. Rec #*: 87654   *Client Room*: 455W
Date: 1/31/11   *Time*: 3:06 PM   *Physician*: Dr. Woodard

S: *Client expressed pleasure with adaptations to prosthetic leg fasteners made this date, stating "this will work."*

O: *Client participated in OT session in rehab gym for adaptations necessary to don/doff prosthesis. Client sit ↔ stand Ⓘ from w/c while keeping one hand on walker for support. Client positioned prosthetic leg and attempted to fasten straps. Client needed mod Ⓐ in fastening of straps, Ⓘ in undoing of straps to doff prosthesis. Adaptations of prosthetic leg harness completed this date.*

A: *Inability to don prosthesis Ⓘ currently limits Ⓘ with dressing, toileting, and functional mobility for IADLs. Client would benefit from additional skilled instruction in use of pulley-like fasteners installed this date on prosthesis to allow one-handed closure.*

P: *Pt. to be seen one more session prior to discharge home tomorrow for skilled instruction in donning prosthesis.*

Joanie W, OTR/L

CONTACT NOTE: SAFETY

Occupational Therapy Note
Date: 4/22/11   *Time*: 10:15 AM

S: *Client reports ↓ activity tolerance and ↑ shortness of breath with exertion. Client reports feeling ok about asking nursing for Ⓐ c̄ dressing, but has urgent incontinence and cannot always wait for Ⓐ to manage O_2 cord to toilet.*

O: *Client participated in OT session in room to assess safety during toileting.*
     Cognition: *WFL; no deficits*
     Functional Mobility: *Client uses walker, has difficulty managing O_2 cord, requires SBA for safety.*
     Upper Extremity Strength: *WNL; client fatigues c̄ use of UE.*
     ADLs: *CGA for clothing management c̄ toileting. Mobility during toileting and dressing requires min Ⓐ for O_2 cord management and safety. Client dresses with mod Ⓐ due to ↓ activity tolerance, and needs to stop p̄ 5 minutes dressing activity.*

A: *Client at risk for falls due to inability to manage O_2 cord during functional mobility to toilet. Client would benefit from adaptive equipment and techniques to toilet with ↑ Ⓘ as well as instruction in energy conservation techniques and ↑ activity tolerance for ADL tasks.*

P: *Client will be seen 2x/wk. for 1 week in order to ↑ Ⓘ and safety in toileting.*

Paige R, OTR/L

Contact Note: Splint

Occupational Therapy Note

Date: *10/20/11*   ***Time***: *3:00 pm*

S: *Mr. J stated that the pain in his right wrist and thumb was "not as bad as it was 2 weeks ago." He reported that his splint is rubbing a calcium deposit on the dorsum of his hand and that he is not wearing the splint at work during the day. He also reported feeling pain during treatment with movement of the Ⓡ thumb and that ice and iontophoresis ↓ pain.*

O: *Mr. J arrived at clinic wearing forearm-based thumb spica splint. Upon removal of splint, wrist appeared slightly swollen.*

     AROM: Wrist flexion ~25%   Wrist extension <25%

              Thumb flexion and extension ~25%

     Mr. J tolerated ~3 minutes friction massage over abductor pollicis longus and extensor pollicis brevis tendons. Ice applied for 5 minutes; Mr. J instructed in using ice at home and at work to ↓ pain by ↓ inflammation of tendons. Splint reformed to eliminate rubbing on dorsum of hand, and Mr. J instructed in wearing schedule at work. HEP modified and Mr. J demonstrated new procedures correctly.

A: *Swelling ↓ since last tx. session shows good progress. Wrist and thumb AROM are ~50% below functional limits due to pain upon movement. Limited AROM & pain are causing functional problems in the work environment. Ice and iontophoresis ↓ pain & therefore ↑ functional ability c̄ Ⓡ hand. Splint reconstruction will also contribute to ↓ pain. Mr. J would benefit from continued skilled OT to ↓ pain, ↑ AROM, ↑ ability to use Ⓡ hand at work.*

P: *Continue to see Mr. J 2x/wk. for the following:*

    ❖ *Ice & iontophoresis to ↓ pain in Ⓡ hand and wrist.*

    ❖ *Friction massage to ↓ inflammation and ↑ AROM in Ⓡ wrist and thumb.*

    ❖ *Re-evaluation of splint for fit and use after reconstruction.*

    ❖ *Re-evaluation of effectiveness and compliance of HEP.*

    ❖ *To achieve goal of ↓ pain in Ⓡ wrist and hand for use in functional activity at work and home.*

Mark S, OTR/L

References

American Academy of Professional Coders. (2009). *ICD-10 implementation date announced.* Retrieved from http://news.aapc. com/index.php/2009/01/icd-10-date-announced/

American Health Information Management Association. (2009). *AHIMA history.* Retrieved from http://www.ahima.org/ about/history.aspx

American Medical Association. (2009). *CPT code/relative value search.* Retrieved from https://catalog.ama-assn.org/Catalog/ cpt/cpt_search.jsp

American Occupational Therapy Association. (1989). Uniform terminology for occupational therapy—second edition. *American Journal of Occupational Therapy, 43*(12), 808-815.

American Occupational Therapy Association. (2006a). *AOTA's centennial vision.* Retrieved from http://www.aota.org/News/ Centennial/Background/36516.aspx?FT=.pdf

American Occupational Therapy Association. (2006b). Guidelines to the occupational therapy code of ethics. *American Journal of Occupational Therapy, 60*(6), 652-658.

American Occupational Therapy Association. (2007a). Accreditation standards for a doctoral-degree-level education program for the occupational therapist. *American Journal of Occupational Therapy, 61*(6), 641-651.

American Occupational Therapy Association. (2007b). Accreditation standards for a master's-degree-level educational program for the occupational therapist. *American Journal of Occupational Therapy, 61*(6), 652-661.

American Occupational Therapy Association. (2007c). Accreditation standards for an educational program for the occupational therapy assistant. *American Journal of Occupational Therapy, 61*(6), 662-671.

American Occupational Therapy Association. (2007d). *OT/OTA student supervision & Medicare requirements.* Retrieved from http://www.aota.org/Educate/EdRes/Fieldwork/StuSuprvsn/38386.aspx

American Occupational Therapy Association. (2008a). Guidelines for documentation of occupational therapy. *American Journal of Occupational Therapy, 62*(6), 684-690.

American Occupational Therapy Association. (2008b). Occupational therapy practice framework: Domain & process, 2nd edition. *American Journal of Occupational Therapy, 62*(6), 625-688.

American Occupational Therapy Association. (2009). Guidelines for supervision, roles, and responsibilities during the delivery of occupational therapy services. *American Journal of Occupational Therapy, 63*(6), 797-803.

American Occupational Therapy Association. (2010a). *Occupational therapy code of ethics and ethics standards (2010).* Retrieved from http://www.aota.org/Practitioners/Ethics/Docs/Standards/38527.aspx

American Occupational Therapy Association. (2010b). *Occupational therapy services in the promotion of psychological and social aspects of mental health.* Retrieved from http://www.aota.org/Practitioners/PracticeAreas/MentalHealth/ Highlights/40878.aspx

American Occupational Therapy Association. (2010c). Scope of practice. *American Journal of Occupational Therapy, 64*(Suppl.), S70-S71. Doi: 10.5014/ajpt.2010.64S70-64S71.

American Occupational Therapy Association. (2010d). *Standards of practice for occupational therapy.* Retrieved from http:// www.aota.org/Practitioners/Official/Standards/36194.aspx

Gateley CA, Borcherding S. *Documentation Manual for Occupational Therapy: Writing SOAP Notes, 3rd Edition* (pp. 211-214)
© 2012 SLACK Incorporated

American Physical Therapy Association. (2010). *Form requirements for the "plan of treatment" for outpatient rehabilitation.* Retrieved from http://www.apta.org/AM/Template.cfm?Section=Home&TEMPLATE=/CM/ContentDisplay.cfm&CONTENTID=30970

Baron, R. (2007). Quality improvement with an electronic health record: Achievable, but not automatic. *Annals of Internal Medicine, 147*(8), 549-552.

Bazyk, S., & Case-Smith, J. (2010). School-based occupational therapy. In J. Case-Smith & J. O'Brien (Eds.), *Occupational therapy for children* (6th ed., pp. 713-743). Maryland Heights, MO: Mosby/Elsevier.

Benemerito, T. (2000). Why you need to know your practice act. *OT Practice, 5*(9), 10.

Berger, S., & Diamant, R. (2005). Documentation. In A. Wagenfeld & J. Kaldenberg (Eds.), *Foundations of pediatric practice for the occupational therapy assistant* (pp. 41-52). Thorofare, NJ: SLACK Incorporated.

Black, T., & Eberhardt, K. (2005). *The occupational therapy assistant: Resources for practice & education.* Bethesda, MD: AOTA Press.

Borcherding, S., & Morreale, M. (2007). *The OTA's guide to writing SOAP notes.* Thorofare, NJ: SLACK Incorporated.

Brachtesende, A. (2005). ICF: The universal translator. *OT Practice, 10*(16), 14-17.

Brennan, C., & Robinson, M. (2006). Documentation: Getting it right to avoid Medicare denials. *OT Practice, 11*(14), 10-15.

Brodnik, M. (2007). The health informatics and information management profession. In M. Abdelhak, S. Grostick, M. Hanken, & E. Jacobs (Eds.), *Health information: Management of a strategic resource* (3rd ed., pp. 42-61). St. Louis, MO: Saunders/Elsevier.

Brown, C. (2009). Ecological models in occupational therapy. In E. B. Crepeau, E. S. Cohn, & B. A. Boyt Schell (Eds.), *Willard & Spackman's occupational therapy* (11th ed., pp. 435-445). Philadelphia, PA: Lippincott Williams & Wilkins.

Carter, J. (2008). *Electronic health records: A guide for clinicians and administrators* (2nd ed.). Philadelphia, PA: ACP Press.

Centers for Medicare & Medicaid Services. (2009a). *Certification & compliance: Overview.* Retrieved from http://www.cms.gov/CertificationandComplianc/01_Overview.asp

Centers for Medicare & Medicaid Services. (2009b). *Medicare & you.* Retrieved from http://www.q1medicare.com/pics/ContentPics/MedicareAndYou2009_10050.pdf

Center for Medicare & Medicaid Services. (2009c). *Medicare and your mental health benefits.* Retrieved from http://www.medicare.gov/publications/pubs/pdf/10184.pdf

Centers for Medicare & Medicaid Services. (2009d). *Personal health records: Overview.* Retrieved from http://www.cms.gov/PerHealthRecords/

Centers for Medicare & Medicaid Services. (2009e). *Prospective payment systems—General information: Overview.* Retrieved from http://www.cms.gov/prospmedicarefeesvcpmtgen/

Centers for Medicare & Medicaid Services. (2009f). *Therapy services: Overview.* Retrieved from http://www.cms.gov/therapyservices/

Centers for Medicare & Medicaid Services. (2010a). *Inpatient rehabilitation facility PPS: IRF Patient Assessment Instrument.* Retrieved from http://www.cms.gov/InpatientRehabFacPPS/04_IRFPAI.asp

Centers for Medicare & Medicaid Services. (2010b). *Identifiable data files: Long term care Minimum Data Set (MDS).* Retrieved from http://www.cms.gov/IdentifiableDataFiles/10_LongTermCareMinimumDataSetMDS.asp

Chabner, D. (2004). *Medical language instant translator* (2nd ed.). St. Louis, MO: Elsevier.

Chandler, B. (2007). IEP goals, but not an OT goal in sight. *ADVANCE for Occupational Therapy Practitioners, 23*(20), 16-17.

Clark, F., & Bloom, P. (2006). *The centennial vision: A call to action.* Retrieved from http://www.aota.org/News/Centennial/Background/36566.aspx

Creek, J. (2008). Approaches to practice. In J. Creek & L. Lougher (Eds.), *Occupational therapy and mental health* (pp. 3-14). Edinburgh: Churchill Livingstone Elsevier.

Crepeau, E., Boyt Schell, B., & Cohn, E. (2009a). Contemporary occupational therapy practice in the United States. In E. B. Crepeau, E. S. Cohn, & B. A. Boyt Schell (Eds.), *Willard & Spackman's occupational therapy* (11th ed., pp. 216-221). Philadelphia, PA: Lippincott Williams & Wilkins.

Crepeau, E., Boyt Schell, B., & Cohn, E. (2009b). Theory and practice in occupational therapy. In E. B. Crepeau, E. S. Cohn, & B. A. Boyt Schell (Eds.), *Willard & Spackman's occupational therapy* (11th ed., pp. 428-434). Philadelphia, PA: Lippincott Williams & Wilkins.

Darzins, P., Fone S., & Darzins, S. (2006). The International Classification of Functioning, Disability and Health can help to structure and evaluate therapy. *Australian Occupational Therapy Journal, 53,* 127-131.

Davis, J., Zayat, E., Urton, M., Belgum, A., & Hill, M. (2008). Communicating evidence in clinical documentation. *Australian Occupational Therapy Journal, 55,* 249-255.

Diamant, R. B. (2004). Integration of occupational therapy practice framework and international classifications of functioning concepts: Application of role performance in client-centered practice. *WFOT Bulletin, 50*, 24-32.

DiCarlo, T. (2008). Productivity in today's SNF. *ADVANCE for Occupational Therapy Practitioners, 24*(23). Retrieved from http://occupational-therapy.advanceweb.com/editorial/content/editorial.aspx?CC=188048

Dickie, V., Cutchin, M. P., & Humphry, R. (2006). Occupation as a transactional experience: A critique of individualism in occupational science. *Journal of Occupational Science, 13*, 83-93.

Engel, L., Henderson, C., Fergenbaum, J., & Colantonio, A. (2009). Medical record review conduction model for improving interrater reliability of abstracting medical-related information. *Evaluation & the Health Professions, 32*(3), 281-298.

Erickson, M., McKnight, R., & Utzman, R. (2008). *Physical therapy documentation: From examination to outcome.* Thorofare, NJ: SLACK Incorporated.

Ford, E., Menachemi, N., Peterson, L., & Huerta, T. (2009). Resistance is futile: But it is slowing the pace of EHR adoption nonetheless. *Journal of the American Medical Informatics Association, 16*(3), 274-81.

Freedman, S. (2006). Understand the nuances of utilization review and utilization management. *Managed Healthcare Executive.* Retrieved from http://managedhealthcareexecutive.modernmedicine.com/mhe/article/articleDetail.jsp?id=282713

Gagan, M.J. (2009). The SOAP format enhances communication. *Kai Tiaki Nursing New Zealand, 15*(5), 15.

Graham, G., Strouse, K., & Haddad, M. (2007). Classification systems, clinical vocabularies, and terminology. In M. Abdelhak, S. Grostick, M. Hanken, & E. Jacobs (Ed.), *Health information: Management of a strategic resource* (3rd ed., pp. 198-217). St. Louis, MO: Saunders Elsevier.

Haglund, L., & Henriksson, C. (2003). Concepts in occupational therapy in relation to the ICF. *Occupational Therapy International, 10*(4), 253-268.

Hartmann, K. (2008). Practice perks: The role of Official Documents. *OT Practice, 13*(22), 10.

Hemmingsson, H., & Jonsson, H. (2005). An occupational perspective on the concept of participation in the International Classification of Functioning, Disability and Health—Some critical remarks. *American Journal of Occupational Therapy, 59*(5), 569-576.

Hemphill-Pearson, B. (Ed.). (2008). *Assessments in occupational therapy mental health.* Thorofare, NJ: SLACK Incorporated.

Holmquist, B. (2004). Incorporating the occupational therapy practice framework into a mental health practice setting. *Mental Health Special Interest Section Quarterly, 27*(2), 1-4.

Hussey, S., Sabonis-Chafee, B., & O'Brien, J. (2007). *Introduction to occupational therapy.* St. Louis, MO: Mosby Elsevier.

Jackson, L. (2007). *Occupational therapy services for children and youth under IDEA.* Bethesda, MD: AOTA Press.

Joint Commission on the Accreditation of Healthcare Organizations. (2009). *The official "do not use" list of abbreviations.* Retrieved from http://www.jointcommission.org/Do_Not_Use_List_of_Abbreviations/

King, P., & Olson, D. (2009). Work. In E. B. Crepeau, E. S. Cohn, & B. A. Boyt Schell (Eds.), *Willard & Spackman's occupational therapy* (11th ed., pp. 615-632). Philadelphia, PA: Lippincott Williams & Wilkins.

Koval, K. J., & Cooley, M. R. (2005). Clinical pathway after hip fracture. *Disability and Rehabilitation, 27*(18-19), 1053-1060.

Lohman, H., & Lamb, A. (2009). Payment for services in the United States. In E. B. Crepeau, E. S. Cohn, & B. A. Boyt Schell (Eds.), *Willard & Spackman's occupational therapy* (11th ed., pp. 949-963). Philadelphia, PA: Lippincott Williams & Wilkins.

Lohr, S. (2009, March 1). How to make electronic medical records a reality. *The New York Times.* Retrieved from http://www.nytimes.com

Mathieson, K., & Hahn, C. (2010). Qualified mental health professions. *ADVANCE for Occupational Therapy Practitioners, 26*(11), 10.

Merriam-Webster. (2003). *Merriam-Webster's collegiate dictionary* (11th ed.). Springfield, MA: Author.

Moyers, P., & Dale, L. (2007). *The guide to occupational therapy practice* (2nd ed.). Bethesda, MD: AOTA Press.

Mulligan, S. (2003). *Occupational therapy evaluation for children: A pocket guide.* Philadelphia, PA: Lippincott Williams & Wilkins.

Myers, C., Stephens, L., & Tauber, S. (2010). Early intervention. In J. Case-Smith & J. O'Brien (Eds.), *Occupational therapy for children* (6th ed., pp. 681-709). Maryland Heights, MO: Mosby/Elsevier.

Myers, T. (Ed.). (2009). *Mosby's dictionary of medicine, nursing & health professions.* St. Louis, MO: Mosby/Elsevier.

National Endowment for Financial Education. (2006). *Understanding private health insurance.* Retrieved from http://health-insuranceinfo.net/managing-medical-bills/Understand_Private_Health_Insurance.pdf

O' Harrow, R., Jr. (2009, August 21). U.S. to dole out $1.2 billion for health records technology. *The Washington Post.* Retrieved from http://www.washingtonpost.com

Pape, L., & Ryba, K. (2004). *Practical considerations for school-based occupational therapists.* Bethesda, MD: AOTA Press.

Paterson, C. (2008). A short history of occupational therapy in psychiatry. In J. Creek & L. Lougher (Eds.), *Occupational therapy and mental health* (pp. 3-14). Edinburgh, UK: Churchill Livingstone Elsevier.

Price, P. (2009). The therapeutic relationship. In E. B. Crepeau, E. S. Cohn, & B. A. Boyt Schell (Eds.), *Willard & Spackman's occupational therapy* (11th ed., pp. 328-341). Philadelphia, PA: Lippincott Williams & Wilkins.

Roach, W., Hoban, R., Broccolo, B., Roth, A., & Blanchard, T. (2006). *Medical records and the law* (4th ed.). Sudbury, MA: Jones and Bartlett Publishers.

Robinson, M. (2007). Medicare 101: Understanding the basics. *OT Practice, 12*(2), CE1-CE8.

Roberts, P., & Evenson, M. (2009). Settings providing medical and psychiatric services. In E. B. Crepeau, E. S. Cohn, & B. A. Boyt Schell (Eds.), *Willard & Spackman's occupational therapy* (11th ed., pp. 1074-1079). Philadelphia, PA: Lippincott Williams & Wilkins.

Rosa, S. (2009). Client-centered collaboration. In E. B. Crepeau, E. S. Cohn, & B. A. Boyt Schell (Eds.), *Willard & Spackman's occupational therapy* (11th ed., pp. 286-290). Philadelphia, PA: Lippincott Williams & Wilkins.

Sames, K. (2009). Documentation in practice. In E. B. Crepeau, E. S. Cohn, & B. A. Boyt Schell (Eds.), *Willard & Spackman's occupational therapy* (11th ed., pp. 403-410). Philadelphia, PA: Lippincott Williams & Wilkins.

Sames, K. (2010). *Documenting occupational therapy practice* (2nd ed.). Upper Saddle River, NJ: Pearson.

Scott, R. (2006). *Legal aspects of documenting patient care for rehabilitation professionals.* Sudbury, MA: Jones and Bartlett Publishers.

Shipp, M., & Havard, A. (2006). Documenting driver rehabilitation services and outcomes. In J. M. Pellerito, Jr. (Ed.), *Driver rehabilitation and community mobility.* St. Louis, MO: Elsevier Mosby.

Slater, D. (2006). The ethics of productivity. *OT Practice, 11*(19), 17-20.

Snow, K. (2009). *People first language.* Retrieved from http://www.disabilityisnatural.com/images/PDF/pfl09.pdf

Social Security Administration. (2009). *What is Medicaid?* Retrieved from http://www.socialsecurity.gov/disabilityresearch/wi/medicaid.htm

Stephens, L., & Tauber, S. (2005). Early intervention. In J. Case-Smith (Ed.), *Occupational therapy for children* (5th ed., pp. 771-793). St. Louis, MO: Elsevier Mosby.

Tickle-Degnen, L. (2009). Evidence-based practice. In E. B. Crepeau, E. S. Cohn, & B. A. Boyt Schell (Eds.), *Willard & Spackman's occupational therapy* (11th ed., pp. 291-302). Philadelphia, PA: Lippincott Williams & Wilkins.

Torrey, T. (2011). *What are CPT codes? Do CPT codes affect your health care?* Retrieved from http://patients.about.com/od/costsconsumerism/a/cptcodes.htm

Tripicchio, B., Bykerk, K., Wegner, C., & Wegner, J. (2009). Increasing patient participation: The effects of training physical and occupational therapists to involve geriatric patients in the concerns-clarification and goal-setting processes. *Journal of Physical Therapy Education, 23*(1), 55-63.

Uniform Data System for Medical Rehabilitation. (2010). *About the FIM System®.* Retrieved from http://www.udsmr.org/WebModules/FIM/Fim_About.aspx

U.S. Department of Education. (2006). *IDEA regulations: Individualized Education Program (IEP).* Retrieved from http://idea.ed.gov/explore/view/p/%2Croot%2Cdynamic%2CTopicalBrief%2C10%2C

U.S. Department of Education. (2010). *Model form: Individualized Education Program.* Retrieved from http://idea.ed.gov/download/modelform1_IEP.pdf

U.S. Department of Health & Human Services. (2006). *HIPAA security guidance.* Retrieved from http://controller.ucsf.edu/capital/files/HIPAA_Security_Guidance.pdf

U.S. Department of Health & Human Services. (2009). *What is the difference between Medicare and Medicaid?* Retrieved from http://answers.hhs.gov/questions/3094

Villemaire, D., & Villemaire, L. (2001). *Grammar and writing skills for the health professional.* Albany, NY: Delmar.

Walker, J., Ahern, D., Le, L., & Delbanco, T. (2009). Insights for internists: "I want the computer to know who I am." *Journal of General Internal Medicine, 24*(6), 727-732.

Weir, C., & Nebeker, J. (2007). Critical issues in an electronic documentation system. *AMIA 2007 Symposium Proceedings,* 786-790.

World Health Organization. (2001). *International classification of functioning, disability and health (ICF).* Geneva, Switzerland: Author.

World Health Organization. (2002). *Towards a common language for functioning, disability and health: ICF.* Geneva, Switzerland: Author. Retrieved from http://www.who.int/classifications/icf/training/icfbeginnersguide.pdf

World Health Organization. (2009). *International statistical classification of diseases and related health problems: 10th revision.* Retrieved from http://apps.who.int/classifications/apps/icd/icd10online/

Appendix
Suggestions for Completing the Worksheets

In this appendix, we will offer suggestions for completing the worksheets throughout this manual. As a student or new therapist using this manual, you can work your way through the exercises and check your work against those in this appendix. Remember that your answer can be different and still be correct, as long as it contains the essential elements. As long as your information and protocol are correct, you should not sacrifice your own writing style to be more like someone else's.

SOAP notes are very difficult to write if there is no treatment session about which to write. Although there are many examples in this manual, there is no substitute for observing or working with actual clients. Only then will you be able to translate your treatment session onto paper in a meaningful way.

CHAPTER 4

WORKSHEET 4-1: AVOIDING COMMON DOCUMENTATION ERRORS

1. Pt. stated my head really hurts this morning.
   Pt. stated, "My head really hurts this morning."
2. Resident reported "her right hand is working better today."
   Resident reported her right hand is working better today.
3. Student used right hand to cut with scissors. Student then switches to left hand for coloring tasks. Student did not demonstrate consistent hand preference.
   Student used right hand to cut with scissors. Student then switched to left hand for coloring task. Student did not demonstrate consistent hand preference.
4. The client's expressed excitement about the upcoming visit to the mall.
   The clients expressed excitement about the upcoming visit to the mall.
5. An occupational therapy referral was recieved from the childs' teacher.
   An occupational therapy referral was received from the child's teacher.
6. The child was unable to button their coat.
   The child was unable to button her coat.
7. The resident's were all in the dinning room weighting for there meal.
   The residents were all in the dining room waiting for their meal.
8. Client demonstrated appropriate social interaction by responding your welcome to another group member.
   Client demonstrated appropriate social interaction by responding "You're welcome" to another group member.
9. Pt. required moderate assistance to use dominate right hand in hygeine tasks.
   Pt. required moderate assistance to use dominant right hand in hygiene tasks.

Gateley CA, Borcherding S. *Documentation Manual for Occupational Therapy: Writing SOAP Notes, 3rd Edition* (pp. 215-236)
© 2012 SLACK Incorporated

10. Client does not demonstrate awareness of the affect of his mood on other member's of the group.
    Client does not demonstrate awareness of the effect of his mood on other members of the group.

11. Pt. expressed intrest in getting dressed. Pt required verbal cues when doning pullover shirt to utilize adaptive teckniques due to right rotary cup injury.
    Pt. expressed interest in getting dressed. Pt. required verbal cues when donning pullover shirt to utilize adaptive techniques due to right rotator cuff injury.

12. The ot noticed assymetry in the childs sitting posture. Parents reports that the client is unable to sit independantly.
    The OT noticed asymmetry in the child's sitting posture. Parents reported that the client is unable to sit independently.

13. The OTR preformed a Cognitive Test on the client.
    The OTR performed a cognitive test on the client.

14. The Doctor called to check on the Patients status.
    The doctor called to check on the patient's status.

15. Client demonstrated poor judgement by attempting to stand up without their walker.
    Client demonstrated poor judgment by attempting to stand up without his walker.

16. Pt. had right arm imobilized due to a clavical fracture.
    Pt. had right arm immobilized due to a clavicle fracture.

17. Client required several breif rest brakes during ADL's.
    Client required several brief rest breaks during ADLs.

18. The clinic employs three otr's and two ota's.
    The clinic employs three OTRs and two OTAs.

19. The students principle stated Jimmy is disruptive at school.
    The student's principal stated, "Jimmy is disruptive at school."

20. A child at this age should be able to dress themselves.
    A child at this age should be able to dress herself.

21. The childrens' mother has difficulty keeping all they're appointment's.
    The children's mother has difficulty keeping all their appointments.

22. Client needed a visual aide to help them learn how to preform self-catherization.
    Client needed a visual aid to help him learn how to perform self-catheterization.

Worksheet 4-2: Using Abbreviations

1. Client c/o pain in Ⓡ MCP joint p̄ ~15 min PROM.
   Client complained of pain in the right metacarpophalangeal joint after approximately 15 minutes of passive range of motion.

2. Pt. A&OX4.
   The client was oriented to person, place, time, and situation.

3. Client transferred w/c → mat c̄ sliding board & max Ⓐ X 2.
   Client transferred from his wheelchair to the mat using a sliding board and maximum assistance of two people.

4. 1° dx Ⓛ BKA, 2° dx COPD, CHF, DM, & PVD.
   Primary diagnosis is left below-the-knee amputation. Secondary diagnoses are chronic obstructive pulmonary disease, congestive heart failure, diabetes mellitus, and peripheral vascular disease.

5. Pt. is s/p Ⓡ THR. Orders received for OT 2x/day for ADLs & IADLs, TTWB Ⓡ LE.
   Patient is status post right total hip replacement. Orders received for occupational therapy two times per day for activities of daily living and instrumental activities of daily living. Toe-touch weightbearing restriction for right lower extremity.

6. Client has thirty degrees of passive range of motion in the left distal interphalangeal joint, which is within functional limits.
   30° PROM in Ⓛ DIP is WFL.

7. Client is able to put on her socks with standby assistance, but requires moderate assistance with putting on and taking off left shoe.

   Client dons socks SBA but requires mod Ⓐ to don & doff Ⓛ shoe.

8. The client requires contact guard assistance for balance during her morning dressing, which she performs while sitting on the edge of her bed.

   CGA required for balance for AM dressing EOB.

9. The patient participated in a bedside evaluation of activities of daily living. She was able to perform bed mobility with moderate assistance, but she needed maximum assistance to put on her adult undergarment. She was able to go from a supine position to a sitting position with minimum assistance and from a sitting position to a standing position with moderate assistance.

   Pt. participated in bedside ADL eval. Mod Ⓐ for bed mobility, max Ⓐ to don undergarment. Supine → sit min Ⓐ and sit → stand mod Ⓐ.

10. The resident came to the occupational therapy clinic via wheelchair escort. The resident was observed to lean toward his left. The resident needed verbal cues and minimum assistance in positioning his body in the wheelchair to maintain midline orientation and symmetrical posture. The resident transferred from his wheelchair to the toilet with moderate assistance of one person to help him keep his balance using a standing pivot transfer. He needed verbal cues and visual feedback from a mirror to maintain upright posture.

    Resident to OT via w/c escort. Resident leans Ⓛ and needs verbal cues, visual feedback from mirror, and min physical Ⓐ to maintain symmetrical posture in midline. Standing pivot transfer w/c → toilet mod Ⓐ for balance.

11. The veteran participated in an evaluation in his room to determine relevant client factors. The veteran's short-term memory was three out of three for immediate recall, one out of three after 1 minute, and zero out of three with verbal cues after 5 minutes. The left upper extremity shoulder flexion was a grade of 4, shoulder extension was a grade of 4, elbow flexion was a grade of 4, elbow extension was a grade of 4, wrist flexion was a grade of 4 minus, wrist extension was a grade of 4 minus, and grip strength was 8 pounds. The left upper extremity light touch was intact. The right upper extremity muscle grades and sensation were within functional limits.

    Veteran participated in eval. of client factors seated in w/c. Short-term memory 3/3 immediate recall, 1/3 after 1 minute, 0/3 c̄ verbal cues p̄ 5 min. Ⓛ shoulder and elbow strength grade 4, wrist strength 4-, grip strength 8#. Light touch intact. Ⓡ UE strength and sensation WFL.

Chapter 5

Worksheet 5-1: Identifying the Contributing Factors

1. Area of Occupation = Work
   Consumer is unable to sustain employment longer than 2 weeks due to:
   - *Use of inflammatory language at work.*
   - *Aggressive behaviors on the job.*
   - *Need for frequent redirection to task.*
   - *Drug-seeking behaviors at work.*
   - *Inability to plan and sequence a task.*
   - *Inattention to social cues and personal hygiene.*
   - *Arriving late 3 to 4 times weekly following nightly alcohol use.*
   - *Lack of reliable daycare.*

2. Area of Occupation = ADLs
   Veteran needs 1 ½ hours to complete grooming tasks due to:
   - *Motor planning deficits.*
   - *SOB on exertion and need for frequent rest breaks to regain O₂ saturation.*
   - *<5 minutes activity tolerance before needing rest breaks.*
   - *Inability to sequence the task.*
   - *Slowness in locating items needed for grooming due to low vision.*

- *Intention tremors and rigidity 2° Parkinson's Disease.*
- *Decreased fine motor manipulation in Ⓛ UE.*
- *Muscle weakness and limited AROM in Ⓑ UEs.*

3. Area of Occupation = Education
   Child is unable to complete grade-appropriate written worksheets due to:
   - *Increased tone in Ⓑ hands 2° to cerebral palsy.*
   - *Attention span <2 minutes for seated classroom tasks due to sensory-seeking behaviors.*
   - *Mod verbal cues required to sequence multi-step directions.*
   - *Deficits in figure-ground visual perceptual skills.*
   - *Difficulty holding pencil due to multiple joint contractures related to Juvenile Rheumatoid Arthritis.*
   - *Visual motor deficits.*

WORKSHEET 5-2: WRITING FUNCTIONAL PROBLEM STATEMENTS

1. The client has an acquired injury to his brain. As a result, he is not able to pay attention to task for very long at a time, and he is having trouble completing his morning routine. Usually he can pay attention to what he is doing for about 2 minutes, and needs to be redirected back to the task after that.
   <3 minute attention span 2° ABI interferes with ability to complete ADL tasks.
   or
   Client requires verbal cues to stay on task after ~ 2 minutes of ADL tasks.

2. The child is having trouble in school because she has difficulty staying within the lines when she is writing. She habitually grips her pencil in a gross grasp, although with help (someone's hand placed over hers) she can hold it with her thumb and two fingers.
   Child needs HOH Ⓐ to hold pencil in tripod pinch for writing tasks at school.
   or
   Inability to maintain tripod pinch unassisted limits child's ability to stay within the lines during writing tasks at school.

3. The resident is not very cognitively aware. About 40% of the time she has trouble figuring out what to do first if she has to complete a self-care task, and she doesn't remember what she has just been told.
   Resident needs mod verbal cues in ADL tasks due to ↓ ability to sequence steps of task.
   or
   Memory and sequencing deficits result in safety concerns during ADL tasks.

4. Mr. J has recently sustained a Ⓡ CVA. His Ⓛ arm is flaccid and he forgets that it is there. He needs physical and verbal help with ADL tasks about 60% of the time.
   Client requires max Ⓐ to dress upper body due to flaccid Ⓛ UE and Ⓛ side neglect.
   or
   Flaccidity in Ⓛ UE & Ⓛ UE neglect result in max Ⓐ for grooming and hygiene.

5. The consumer has had trouble finding a job. His appearance is unkempt and he has a strong body odor, neither of which seem troubling to him.
   Inattention to personal hygiene interferes with consumer's ability to find employment.
   or
   Consumer has difficulty finding employment due to unkempt appearance and inattention to personal hygiene.

6. The client is unable to transfer safely w/c ↔ toilet without someone to remind him that he needs to follow his total hip precautions.
   Client requires SBA w/c ↔ toilet due to unfamiliarity with hip precautions.
   or
   Unfamiliarity with hip precautions results in need for SBA to follow hip precautions when toileting following recent THR.

Chapter 6

Worksheet 6-1: Choosing Goals for Medical Necessity

- **Problem**: Client unable to perform sewing due to 2+/5 strength in Ⓡ hand musculature.
    - **LTG**:   Client will perform embroidery Ⓘ for 20 minutes within 8 weeks.
    - **STG**:   In order to ↑ performance of embroidery, client will use needle continuously for 5 minutes within 2 weeks.

Other possible problem statements:

- *Problem*: *Client unable to handle small items needed for grooming due to 2+ strength in Ⓡ hand musculature.*
    - *LTG*: *Client will complete grooming activities Ⓘ within 1 month.*
    - *STG*: *Client will remove lid from toothpaste with min verbal cues for adaptive technique within 2 weeks.*

- *Problem*: *Client unable to write >5 minutes due to 2+ strength in her Ⓡ hand musculature.*
    - *LTG*: *Client will write for 15 minutes with one rest break using adaptive pencil grip within 1 month.*
    - *STG*: *Client will sign first name within 1 week using adaptive pencil grip.*

- *Problem*: *Client unable to fasten ½" buttons due to 2+ strength in Ⓡ hand.*
    - *LTG*: *Client will fasten all buttons on shirt independently.*
    - *STG*: *Within 1 week, client will fasten 3 buttons on shirt using button hook with min Ⓐ.*

Worksheet 6-2: Evaluating Goal Statements

1. By the time of discharge in 2 weeks, client will dress himself with min Ⓐ for balance using a sock aid and reacher while sitting in w/c.
   This goal has all of the necessary COAST components.

2. Client will tolerate 10 minutes of treatment daily.
   This goal lacks an occupation, an assistance level, and a time frame. In addition, the behavior (tolerating treatment) is not useful because it is not something that the client needs to do after discharge. *Client will complete 10 minutes of grooming/hygiene activity with SBA and no rest break within 1 week.*

3. Client will demonstrate increased coping skills when communicating with her daughter within 2 weeks.
   "Coping skills" is far too broad. The coping skill(s) in question need to be specified as well as a way to measure those skills. For example: *By next group session, client will verbalize 2 anger management strategies that can be used when she experiences frustration during interaction with family members.*

4. Client will demonstrate 15 minutes of activity tolerance without rest breaks using Ⓑ UEs in order to complete ADL tasks before breakfast each morning.
   This goal lacks an assistance level and a time frame, and it needs to be turned around to focus on the occupation rather than the specific condition. *By 9/17/2011, client will complete basic ADLs with supervision in <15 minutes without rest breaks each morning before breakfast.*

5. OT will teach lower body dressing using a reacher, dressing stick, and sock aide within 3 treatment sessions.
   Most importantly, this goal is not client-centered. *Client will complete lower body dressing with SBA using reacher, dressing stick, and sock aide within 3 treatment sessions.* **(Remember, what the OT does is the <u>intervention</u>, not the goal.)**

6. Patient will demonstrate ability to balance his checkbook.
   This goal lacks an assistance level, a specific condition, and a time frame. *Within 4 weeks, patient independently will balance checkbook using calculator with no mathematical errors.*

WORKSHEET 6-3: WRITING CLIENT-CENTERED, OCCUPATION-BASED, MEASURABLE GOALS

1. Shontelle is not able to attend to task for more than a few minutes, which makes IADL activities difficult for her. Since she likes to cook and plans to return to cooking after discharge, you have been working with her in the kitchen. You would like to see her able to attend to task for 10 minutes by the time she is discharged next week. Write a goal that addresses Shontelle's attention span during cooking.
   Client will complete cooking activity with supervision, maintaining attention to task at least 10 minutes without redirection within 1 week.
   or
   Within 3 treatment sessions, client will complete cooking activity with supervision, attending to task at least 10 minutes with 2 or fewer verbal cues for redirection.

2. Now write a goal for Shontelle to be able to follow directions so that she can read the back of a boxed meal, and eventually a recipe, when she is cooking.
   Client will complete a cooking activity c̄ min Ⓐ to follow 3-step written direction within 3 treatment sessions.
   or
   Client will follow simple recipe independently within 1 week.

3. Bill is having trouble dressing himself after his stroke. You have been teaching him an over-the-head method for putting on his shirt, and have given him a buttonhook to use. Write a dressing goal for Bill.
   Client will don shirt with modified Ⓘ using over-the-head method and a button hook within 2 tx. sessions.
   or
   After skilled instruction, client will dress upper body with modified independence using one-handed techniques and adaptive equipment within 1 week.

4. Abigail is very weak, and she wants to be able to go back to work as a receptionist. She also wants to be able to care for her 4-month-old child. Write a goal that addresses her activity tolerance during an occupation-based activity.
   Client will complete simulated infant-bathing activity with SBA, standing for at least 10 minutes, by discharge in 2 weeks.
   or
   Within 1 week, client independently will complete seated work-simulation tasks using computer, telephone, and desk-top office supplies for 20 minutes without rest breaks.

5. Rashad wants to live independently in the community, but lacks basic money management skills. Write a goal for Rashad to improve his money management skills.
   Client will make change Ⓘ from $1.00 correctly 3/3 tries within 2 weeks.
   or
   With minimal verbal cues, client will select ads from the newspaper for an apartment that rents for less than 1/3 of his regular monthly income within 3 weeks.

6. Kylie has become increasingly more depressed over the past several weeks and was admitted after a suicide attempt. You estimate that you will have her in group for 1 week. You would like to see her mood change in that week. Write an occupation-based goal that will indicate an improved mood.
   Within 1 week, client will spontaneously follow her daily schedule, as demonstrated by attending at least 3 scheduled activities per day.
   or
   Client spontaneously will verbalize an interest in at least one future activity within the next 2 days.

CHAPTER 7

WORKSHEET 7-1: WRITING CONCISE, COHERENT "S" STATEMENTS

1. Mrs. P is recovering from a total hip replacement. During a treatment session, she makes the following statements:
   - "I used that dressing stick and sock aid like you showed me to get dressed without bending down this morning."
   - "My hip doesn't hurt when I stand up or sit down, especially with that new toilet seat you got for me."
   - "It's getting easier for me to get dressed now."
   - "My daughter said they delivered all that bathroom equipment to her house yesterday."

S: *Client reports using adaptive equipment to don pants and socks while maintaining hip precautions without difficulty. She has not c/o pain with transfers using raised toilet seat. Bathroom equipment ordered by OT last week has been delivered to daughter's home.*

2. Ryan is a 14-year-old recently admitted to an inpatient adolescent psychiatric unit following an unsuccessful suicide attempt by overdose with his mother's sleeping pills. During a group session he makes the following comments:
   - "I have nothing to live for."
   - "I don't have any friends."
   - "My family would be better off without me anyway."
   - "The teachers at my school all hate me."
   - "Maybe next time I should do it right and just use a gun!"

S: *Client reports a lack of self-worth in both family and school situations and states that he does not have any friends. He continues to express suicidal ideation and suggested that he may use a gun in a future suicide attempt.*

WORKSHEET 7-2: CHOOSING A SUBJECTIVE STATEMENT

1. Client was very cooperative and engaged in social conversation throughout the tx. session.
   Even though the client may have been cooperative, and even though it may have been important in this treatment session, it is an assessment of the situation, and does not belong in the "S" category of the note. The client's social conversation might be important in some situations. However, there is a better choice for this particular note.

2. Client remarked that her grandson will be coming to visit later in the week, and that she will be very glad to see him.
   In this instance, a pending visit by the client's grandson is not really relevant to the treatment session or to how the client sees her progress. It might be important in another situation. For example, if the client was planning to go live with her grandson after discharge, it might be very relevant and might be a topic the OT wanted to explore further with the client.

3. Client reports that she feels "pretty good" today.
   Feeling "pretty good" today might be important because it might show progress or a change in her condition. In this case, however, it is not the best choice.

4. Client says she has difficulty moving Ⓡ UE, although she does not know why it will not move. She reports, "It really doesn't hurt. It's just tight."
   The client's comments about her upper extremity seem most pertinent to this treatment session. Use of the Ⓡ UE is relevant in all aspects of this treatment session.

5. Nursing staff report client is incontinent at night.
   This information should be documented in the nursing notes. The subjective section of the note is generally used to document the client's views rather than views of the staff, except in rare instances. For example, if nursing staff had reported a safety concern with the client's ability to transfer to the toilet that was inconsistent with client report or OT observation, then that information would be relevant to this session. There is a better choice for this note.

CHAPTER 8

WORKSHEET 8-1: USING CATEGORIES

O: Child participated in 60-minute OT session at daycare to address feeding skills and reach/grasp/release during play. With min Ⓐ for facilitation of movement at elbow, child demonstrated ability to use Ⓛ UE to reach, grasp, and release 5 objects with 1-2 verbal cues per object and restriction of Ⓡ UE movement. Child was able to feed self Ⓘ c̄ ~50% spillage, but demonstrated significant limitations in chewing action p̄ ~3 rotary chews & swallowing ~90% of food s̄ chewing. Child required verbal cues throughout session to maintain attention to task. Child wore soft spica thumb splint for entire session.

Some or all of the following categories might be used to make this note easier to read:
- Ⓛ UE use or reach/grasp/release
- **Feeding**
- **Attention/attention to task/attention span**
- **Splint**

Depending on the categories selected, the note might read like this:

O: *Child participated in 60-minute OT session at daycare to address functional use of Ⓛ UE during play and self-care. Child wore a Ⓛ soft spica thumb splint throughout tx session to facilitate functional grasp patterns.*
Reach/Grasp/Release: With min Ⓐ for facilitation of elbow, child demonstrated ability to use Ⓛ UE to reach, grasp, and release 5 objects with 1-2 verbal cues per object and restriction of Ⓡ UE movement.
Feeding: Child was able to feed self Ⓘ with ~50% spillage, but demonstrated significant limitation in chewing actions with ~3 rotary chews and swallowing ~90% of the food without chewing.
Attention: Child required verbal cues throughout the session to maintain attention to task.

WORKSHEET 8-2: BEING MORE CONCISE

O: Pt. participated in 60-minute OT session bedside to complete morning ADL routine. Pt. ambulated ~36 inches to shower c̄ SBA for safety. Pt. instructed to complete shower while sitting. Pt performed shower c̄ SBA to manage IV line. Pt. able to wash upper and lower body Ⓘ and dry entire body after completing shower. Pt. required ~20 minutes to complete shower. Pt. then ambulated ~36 inches to chair and sat. Pt. needed verbal cues to remain seated while donning underwear and pants. Pt. able to dress upper body Ⓘ and lower body p̄ verbal cues for sitting. Pt. demonstrated good sitting balance, but needed SBA for standing balance. Following shower, client stated he would like to take a nap and was assisted back to bed.

A more concise note might read:

O: *Pt. participated in 60-minute OT session bedside for skilled instruction in self-care activities. Ambulated ~3 ft. to/from shower c̄ SBA to manage IV line while ambulating and showering for 20 minutes. Client showered and dressed c̄ verbal cues to sit for safety. Client demonstrated good sitting balance but required SBA for standing balance. Client returned to bed c̄ SBA at end of session.*
   or
O: *Client participated in 60-minute OT session in room for skilled instruction in safe showering and dressing. Client ambulated ~3' SBA for balance. After verbal cues to sit, client showered for 20 min c̄ SBA to manage IV lines. Client donned shirt Ⓘ seated; client required verbal cues to remain seated when threading underwear and pants over feet.*

WORKSHEET 8-3: BEING SPECIFIC ABOUT ASSIST LEVELS

1. Client completed supine → sit with min Ⓐ; bed → w/c with mod Ⓐ.
   - *Client completed supine → sit with min Ⓐ to initiate activity; bed → w/c with mod Ⓐ for balance.*
   - *Client completed supine → sit with min Ⓐ to pull up using trapeze; bed → w/c with mod Ⓐ to lift body weight.*
   - *Client completed supine → sit with min Ⓐ to sequence movement; bed → w/c with mod Ⓐ for postural control.*

2. Client required SBA in transferring w/c ↔ toilet.
   - *Client required SBA for proper hand placement in transferring w/c ↔ toilet.*
   - *Client required SBA for sequencing in transferring w/c ↔ toilet.*
3. Client retrieved garments from low drawers with min Ⓐ.
   - *Client retrieved garments from low drawers with min Ⓐ to grasp drawer handles.*
   - *Client retrieved garments from low drawers with min Ⓐ to release trigger on reacher.*
   - *Client retrieved garments from low drawers with min Ⓐ to judge HALO placement in space.*
4. Client required max Ⓐ to brush hair.
   - *Client required max Ⓐ to back of head when brushing hair.*
   - *Client required max Ⓐ to flex Ⓡ shoulder past 35° when brushing hair.*
5. Client completed dressing, toileting, and hygiene with min Ⓐ.
   - *Client completed dressing, toileting, and hygiene with min Ⓐ to reach feet.*
   - *Client completed dressing, toileting, and hygiene with min Ⓐ for activities requiring fine motor dexterity.*
   - *Client completed dressing, toileting, and hygiene with min Ⓐ to adhere to hip precautions.*

WORKSHEET 8-4: DE-EMPHASIZING THE TREATMENT MEDIA

1. Client played catch using Ⓑ UEs to facilitate grasp and release patterns.
   Client worked on functional grasp/release patterns needed to manipulate household objects.
2. Resident put dirt into pot to halfway point, added seedling, and filled remainder of pot with dirt transferred by cup. Resident completed 3 more pots while standing 8 minutes before requiring a 5-minute rest. Resident resumed standing position to water completed pots for approximately 5 minutes.
   Resident demonstrated standing tolerance of 13 minutes with a 5-minute break after 8 minutes in order to increase standing needed for ADL tasks.
3. Client painted some suncatchers in crafts group to be able to see that she could do something successfully.
   Client completed a series of quick-success projects to increase self-esteem.

CHAPTER 9

WORKSHEET 9-1: WRITING ABOUT PROBLEMS IN THE ASSESSMENT

1. Client demonstrated difficulty with laundry and cooking tasks due to memory and sequencing deficits.
   Memory & sequencing deficits cause difficulty c̄ home management tasks.
2. Decreased level of arousal noted during morning dressing activities, requiring redirection to task.
   ↓ level of arousal limits client's ability to complete basic ADL tasks.
3. Client unable to follow hip precautions during morning dressing due to memory deficits.
   Memory deficits interfere c̄ client's ability to incorporate hip precautions into basic self-care tasks.
   or
   Memory deficits limit pt.'s ability to follow hip precautions while dressing.
4. Client problem solved poorly while performing lower body dressing, as evidenced by multiple attempts required to button pants and don socks successfully.
   ↓ problem solving limits client's ability to dress herself s̄ Ⓐ and raises safety concerns in all ADL areas.

WORKSHEET 9-2: JUSTIFYING CONTINUED TREATMENT

Yes Evaluation of a client
No   The practice of coordination and self-care skills on a daily basis
Yes Establishing measurable, behavioral, objective, and individualized goals
Yes Developing intervention plans designed to meet established goals

Yes   Analyzing and modifying functional activities through the provision of adaptive equipment or techniques

Yes   Determining that the modified tasks are safe and effective

No   Carrying out a maintenance program

Yes   Teaching the client to use the breathing techniques he has learned while performing ADL activities

Yes   Providing individualized instruction to the client, family, or caregiver

Yes   Modifying the intervention plan based on a re-evaluation

No   Donning/doffing of a client's resting hand splint on a regular schedule throughout the day

Yes   Providing specialized instruction to eliminate limitations in a functional activity

Yes   Developing a home program and instructing caregivers

Yes   Making changes in the environment

Yes   Teaching compensatory skills

No   Gait training

Yes   Adding instruction in lower body dressing techniques to a current ADL program

No   Presenting informational handouts without having the client perform the activity

Yes   Teaching adaptive techniques such as one-handed shoe tying

No   Routine exercise and strengthening programs

WORKSHEET 9-3: WRITING THE ASSESSMENT—ELLIE'S DEVELOPMENT

A: *Infant's inability to right head, roll, or push up to prone ① limits ability to engage in age-appropriate play skills and developmental exploration. Infant's decreased activity tolerance also limits her ability to engage in developmental play activities. Infant shows progress through ability to maintain facilitated positions and decrease in oxygen need. Visual tracking and scanning by turning head indicates visual awareness and orientation and shows good potential for increased interaction with environment. Infant would benefit from continued facilitation of functional mobility during play as well as increasing strength and endurance through activities that stimulate normal development.*
    or

A: *Decreased postural control and need for facilitation of weight shift limits infant's ability to perform early mobility skills needed for play. Limited mobility combined with her tolerance for less than 20 minutes of activity and the need for frequent rest breaks limit her ability to explore her environment and reach developmental milestones at a typical age. Ability to perform transitional movements with facilitation, orientation to black and white design, and ability to track in horizontal plane show good potential for future developmental gains. Infant would benefit from continued OT services to stimulate developmental skills and from parent education in a home program.*

WORKSHEET 9-4: WRITING THE ASSESSMENT—MS. D'S SOCIAL SKILLS

1. What problems do you see in the above "S" and "O"?
   - **Unkempt appearance**
   - **Interrupts when others are talking**
   - **Does not stay on topic of conversation**
2. What areas of occupation do these problems impact?
   - **Social participation**
3. What evidence of progress and/or potential do you see?
   - **Engages in conversation**
   - **States that she understands purpose of the group**
   - **Willingness to attend and participate in group**
   - **Spontaneously shared thoughts and ideas**
4. What would this client benefit from?
   - **Groups that focus on conversational skills**
   - **Skilled instruction in attending to social cues**
   - **ADL activities stressing hygiene and appearance**

5. Write a complete assessment statement for this note.

A: *Client's unkempt appearance, interrupting behaviors, and need for redirection to topic of conversation interfere with her ability to engage in social participation with peers. Her expressed interest in groups and her willingness to engage in conversation and share her ideas show good potential to develop relationships and to express herself verbally in place of acting out. Client would benefit from participating in groups where conversational skills are stressed, from further facilitation of attention to social cues, and from instruction in ADL activities stressing hygiene and appearance.*

CHAPTER 10

WORKSHEET 10-1: COMPLETING THE PLAN FOR ELLIE

P: *Infant to be seen 2x per week for 30 minutes each visit for 3 months for stimulation of normal developmental sequences and facilitation of appropriate movement patterns during play and exploratory activities. Design and modification of home program for parents also planned.*

or

P: *Child will be seen in home twice weekly for 3 months for activities that encourage postural control needed for play and environmental exploration. Sessions to include parent education targeted at facilitating infant's development. Plan to formally reassess infant's developmental level using standardized testing in 3 months.*

WORKSHEET 10-2: COMPLETING THE PLAN FOR MS. D

P: *Client to be seen daily for the next week to ↑ skills needed for social participation in a variety of contexts. Focus will be on development of conversational skills including not interrupting others and staying on topic.*

or

P: *Client to continue social skills group 3x/wk for 1 wk to improve conversational skills. Client will also be given individual feedback daily on her attention to appearance and social cues.*

CHAPTER 11

WORKSHEET 11-1: WRITING PROBLEM STATEMENTS

1. Pt unable to dress LE ⓘ due to trunk instability.
    - **Tell what assist level is needed rather than saying unable to dress ⓘ.**
    - **Say "lower body" rather than LE, since the client is dressing more than just the extremity.**
    - **If there is one particular part of the task that requires assistance, specify that. For example:** *Client needs mod Ⓐ to maintain balance while dressing lower body due to trunk instability.*
2. Child doesn't tolerate very much classroom activity due to ↓ activity tolerance.
    - **Specify how much "very much" is.**
    - **Tell what kind of classroom activity. For example:** *Child tolerates less than 30 minutes of desk work in classroom due to ↓ activity tolerance.*
3. Consumer acts out.
    - **Specify what is meant by "acts out."**
    - **Specify what area of occupation is problematic because of the acting out.**
    - **Specify the contributing factor that is responsible for the acting out. For example:**
        - *Consumer cuts or burns extremities when upset, resulting in frequent emergency room visits and difficulty resolving conflict with spouse.*
        - *Inappropriate verbal and physical actions result in difficulty sustaining friendships.*

WORKSHEET 11-2: WRITING COAST GOALS

1. Client will make a clock independently using the appropriate materials by anticipated discharge in 1 week.
   Client will demonstrate ability to grasp/place/release objects of various sizes needed for IADL activities by assembling a clock ⓘ by anticipated discharge in 1 week.
   or
   Client will demonstrate ability to follow written directions for IADL tasks by assembling a clock from written instructions ⓘ within 1 week.
2. Consumer will stay in his chair without reminders and spend at least 30 minutes lacing the leather billfold during the 45-minute craft group session within 2 weeks.
   Within 2 weeks, client will demonstrate attention to task needed to qualify for sheltered workshop program by staying in his chair without reminders and attending to craft project 30 minutes or more.

WORKSHEET 11-3: SOAPING YOUR NOTE

O   Client supine → sit in bed ⓘ.

O   Client moved kitchen items from counter to cabinet ⓘ using Ⓛ hand.

A   Decreased coordination, strength, sensation, and proprioception in Ⓛ hand create safety risks in home management tasks.

S   Client reports that his fingers are stiff this morning and that he is having trouble handling small items like buttons.

A   ↑ of 15 minutes in activity tolerance for UE activities permits client to prepare a light meal ⓘ.

O   Child participated in 60-minute eval. of hand function in OT clinic.

A   Decreased proprioception and motor planning limit ⓘ in upper body dressing.

P   Continue retrograde massage to Ⓡ hand for edema control.

A   Correct identification of inappropriate positioning 100% of time indicates memory WFL.

S   Client reports that she cannot remember hip precautions.

A   Veteran would benefit from further instruction to incorporate total hip precautions into lower body dressing, bathing, and toileting.

A   Client's improvement with repetition indicates good potential for successful access of augmentative communication device using eye gaze.

O   Client did not make eye contact during group session.

O   Client wrote check for correct amount to pay electric bill with 2 verbal cues.

A   Client's request to take breaks demonstrates awareness of her limitations in endurance.

O   Client completed weight shifts of trunk X 10 in each of anterior, posterior, left, and right lateral directions in preparation for standing to perform IADLs.

A   3+ muscle grade of Ⓡ wrist extension this week shows good progress toward goals.

P   Continue OT 3x/wk. for 2 weeks to address cognitive impairments that impact safe performance of IADLs.

A   Unkempt appearance in mock interview situation indicates poor judgment and self-concept.

WORKSHEET 11-4: WRITING THE "S"—SUBJECTIVE

S: *Client reports arthritis in Ⓡ shoulder and Ⓛ knee, pain on weightbearing. Pain at Ⓡ BKA site 8/10. During transfer, client requested specific adjustments such as sliding board placement, proximity to bed, and approaching from Ⓡ side. Fatigue reported after transfer.*
     or
S: *Pt. reports significant arthritis in Ⓡ shoulder and Ⓛ knee, and prefers to approach transfers from Ⓡ side. Pt. reports, "It hurts to stand on my left leg." Pt. also stated w/c → bed sliding board transfers are the most difficult, and reported fatigue after transfer.*
     or
S: *Client reports arthritis in Ⓡ shoulder and Ⓛ knee and pain weightbearing on Ⓛ LE. Pt. able to verbalize needs regarding transfer (placement of sliding board and approach from affected side). Client reports fatigue after transfer.*

Worksheet 11-5: "O"—Writing Good Opening Lines

1. Client seen in room for 45 minutes for self-care activities.
   - *Client participated in 45-minute OT session in room to increase Ⓘ in ADL activities, to decrease safety concerns during functional mobility for ADLs, and to provide instruction on proper use of adaptive equipment.*
   - *Client participated in 45-minute OT session in hospital room for education on use of adaptive equipment and toilet transfer during morning self-care activities.*
   - *Client participated in 45-minute OT session at bedside for education on safety concerns during ADLs and skilled instruction in use of adaptive equipment.*
   - *Client participated in 45-minute OT session at bedside for skilled instruction in use of adaptive equipment and hip precaution education during performance of morning ADLs and toilet transfers.*

2. Client seen at workshop for 1 hr. to work on job skills.
   - *Client participated in 1-hr. session at workshop to address cognitive, sensory, and bilateral integration barriers to performing work tasks effectively.*
   - *Client participated in 1-hr. session at workshop to work on sequencing, bilateral coordination, concentration, and sensory awareness while completing work task of package handling.*
   - *Client participated in 1-hr. session @ sheltered workshop for skilled instruction in task sequencing, Ⓑ coordination, and techniques to decrease sensory registration to increase attention for job skills.*

3. Client seen bedside for 30 minutes for morning dressing.
   - *Client participated in 30-minute bedside session for morning dressing to improve balance, Ⓑ motor control, functional mobility during ADLs, and safety in order to return home.*
   - *Client participated in 30-minute bedside session to increase balance and Ⓑ motor control for safety during basic ADLs and use of manual w/c.*
   - *Client participated in 30-minute bedside session to enhance balance and Ⓑ motor tasks involving UE to increase safety during dressing and w/c mobility.*

4. Client seen in kitchen for 1 hr. to work on Ⓘ in cooking.
   - *Client participated in 1-hr. session in kitchen to increase dynamic standing balance and increase awareness of affected UE for safety in cooking.*
   - *Client participated in 1-hr. session in kitchen to work on cooking tasks with attention to standing balance, affected UE position, and safety.*
   - *Client participated in 1-hr. session in kitchen for skilled instruction in kitchen safety to improve standing balance and attention to affected UE.*

Worksheet 11-6: "O"—Being Specific About Assist Levels

No   Client required max Ⓐ x 2 bed → bedside commode and bed → w/c; Ⓓ for pericare.
Yes   Child required HOH Ⓐ to stay in the lines when following path with crayon.
Yes   Client needed mod verbal cues to participate in discussion during life skills group.
No   Resident needed min Ⓐ to don sock due to pain.

Worksheet 11-7: Revising the "O"

✦ An opening line is needed, stating where, for how long, and for what purpose the client was seen. One possibility is: *Client participated in 30-minute session in room for skilled instruction in compensatory dressing techniques and evaluation of splinting needs.*

✦ The categories could be reduced to three: toileting, dressing, and splinting evaluation.

✦ It would be helpful to know what part of the task required assistance.

✦ The UE and LE wording is not inclusive enough since the client is dressing the upper and lower body rather than just the extremities.

✦ Under "hand status," there is no functional component, and "index finger greatest amount" is not very informative.

WORKSHEET 11-8: DIFFERENTIATING BETWEEN OBSERVATIONS AND ASSESSMENTS

O Client is unable to don AFO and shoe Ⓘ for ambulation.

A Inability to don AFO and shoe Ⓘ prevent client from ambulating safely around the house for IADL performance in order to live alone.

A Decreased sensory tolerance limits the client's attention to task in the classroom.

O Client required verbal cues to stay on task due to decreased sensory tolerance.

O Client was unable to incorporate breathing and energy conservation techniques, requiring several prompts to complete task.

A Inability to incorporate breathing techniques and energy conservation techniques into basic ADL tasks s̄ verbal prompts limits her ability to live alone Ⓘ p̄ discharge.

1. Client demonstrated difficulty with laundry and cooking tasks due to memory and sequencing deficits.
    - *Decreased memory and sequencing abilities limit client's ability to perform IADL activities such as laundry and cooking tasks.*
    - *Memory and sequencing deficits interfere with client's ability to perform IADLs such as laundry and cooking, and limit her ability to return to an Ⓘ living situation.*
    - *Deficits in memory and sequencing lead to difficulty with IADL tasks such as laundry and cooking tasks necessary for household management.*

2. Client unable to complete homemaking tasks or basic self-care activities independently due to decreased endurance and not following hip precautions.
    - *Decreased endurance and non-adherence to hip precautions limit client's ability to complete homemaking tasks and self-care activities Ⓘ.*
    - *Failure to follow hip precautions and decreased endurance interfere with client's ability to complete homemaking tasks and decrease ability to successfully complete basic self-care activities Ⓘ.*
    - *Decreased endurance and failure to follow hip precautions prevent client from performing homemaking and ADL task Ⓘ and safely.*

3. After the use of behavioral modification techniques, client displayed courteous behavior for the remainder of the treatment session.
    You could take a positive or negative approach to this one:
    - Positive:
        ❖ *Client's ability to behave courteously with the aid of behavioral modification techniques indicates good potential for improving problem behaviors at school.*
        ❖ *Positive response to behavioral modification techniques shows good potential to meet social participation goals.*
    - Negative:
        ❖ *Need for behavioral modification techniques to elicit courteous behavior limits client's ability to interact appropriately with peers in social settings.*
        ❖ *Need for instruction in behavior modification limits his ability to communicate with others effectively in social situations.*

WORKSHEET 11-9: PROBLEMS, PROGRESS, AND REHAB POTENTIAL

Problems: After reading through this note, several problems stood out for this OT:
- **Dynamic sitting balance**
- **Weight shifting**
- **Posture**
- **Transfers**

(The four above are related to safety and functional mobility.)
- **Decreased AROM in Ⓡ UE (mod Ⓐ to reach)**
- **Cognition**

On thinking a little further, she decided that the "cognition" problem might really be one of the following, since he does seem to understand the goal of the activity:

- **Short-term memory**
- **Motor planning**
- **Problem solving**
- **Initiation**

Finally, the OT decided that the problem with initiation is probably some combination of problem solving and motor planning deficits.

Progress/Rehab Potential: Ability to understand the treatment goal

- **The therapist then groups the problems according to the impact they have on the client's occupational performance. She decides that the first three cause difficulty with functional mobility and are of particular concern because they create safety issues. The motor planning and initiation problem is a concern in the area of self-care, as is the problem with decreased AROM of the Ⓡ UE. The need for continual instruction, whether it is a problem with short-term memory or with his ability to problem solve, is likely to require a lot of attention from a caregiver at home. The client does, however, understand why he is doing the task she has given him. As long as the goals are not set too high, he should be able to make good progress in rehabilitation. Her assessment and plan read as follows:**

A: *Deficits in postural control, dynamic sitting balance, and weight shifting raise safety concerns when transferring. ↓ AROM and motor planning ability negatively impact ability to perform self-care tasks. Need for continual instruction for safety will necessitate a high level of caregiver assistance during ADL tasks. Client's ability to understand treatment goal indicates good rehab potential for goals established. Client would benefit from continued skilled instruction in activities to ↑ balance, safe functional mobility, and Ⓘ in ADL tasks.*

P: *Continue tx daily for 3 weeks for skilled instruction in self-care tasks and safe transfers during ADLs. Focus will be on improving level of independence to min Ⓐ or better in order to return home with caregiver assistance. Adaptive equipment needs for home will also be assessed.*

Another OT might assess the situation a little differently. For example:

A: *Deficits in motor planning, movement initiation, cognition, and muscle weakness in Ⓡ UE result in ↓ safety and independence in ADL tasks and functional mobility during ADLs. Good progress noted in improvement in activity tolerance from <1 minute yesterday to >3 minutes today. Client would benefit from skilled OT to increase balance, functional mobility, and grasp/release activities with involved UE in order to ↑ Ⓘ in self-care activities.*

P: *Continue tx. b.i.d for ½-hour sessions for 3 weeks to work on Ⓡ UE movement and cognitive retraining. Sessions will focus on improving independence in grooming, dressing, toileting, and bathing in order to work toward goal of returning home with spouse. Will consult with speech language pathologist regarding short-term memory strategies that can be incorporated during OT sessions.*
    or

A: *Decreased functional use of Ⓡ UE, decreased sitting balance, and difficulty with sequencing and problem solving limit ability to perform ADLs. Increased shoulder flexion and motor planning since initial evaluation and increased understanding of treatment activities indicate good rehab potential. Client would benefit from continued skilled OT to increase functional AROM, exercises in grasp, exercises in weight shifting to improve dynamic sitting balance, and evaluation of both cognitive status and ability to initiate activity in order to increase Ⓘ in ADL tasks.*

P: *Continue b.i.d. for 30 minute sessions for 3 weeks to increase independence with ADLs. Initial sessions to address dynamic sitting balance and functional Ⓡ UE movement in preparation for ADL training.*

Worksheet 11-10: Writing the "A" and "P"—The School Note

Problems:
- Decreased visual tracking and eye convergence
- Low muscle tone/upper body weakness
- Decreased bilateral coordination
- Impaired fine motor skills
- Poor handwriting
- UE weakness
- Proximal instability

Progress/Rehab Potential:
- Improvement in ability to form letters within lines
- 90% accuracy from memory of some letters
- Handwriting improvement

A: *Decreased upper body strength and proximal stability limit the child's ability to use his upper extremities in an accurate and coordinated manner in class. Lack of fine motor and bilateral coordination limit the child's accuracy in schoolwork (including handwriting, art, and play activities). Inaccuracy in visual tracking and eye convergence interfere with ability to form letters and numbers or to complete written work from a book or whiteboard at grade level. Lack of visual tracking and convergence skills also limits ability to perform age-appropriate games safely. Improvement in accuracy of letter formation since last note and ability to remember 6 letter shapes indicate good progress and good potential to meet IEP goals. Child would benefit from continued work on postural stability to support functional UE use, as well as from continued work on visual and motor skills needed for classroom activities.*

P: *Continue OT twice weekly for 30-minute sessions for remainder of school year to improve functional performance in educational activities. Sessions to focus on improving postural control, bilateral coordination, and oculomotor control. Will consult with classroom teacher regarding classwork modifications to accommodate oculomotor deficits.*

Worksheet 11-11: Writing the "A" and "P"—Mr. S's Communication Skills

Problems:
- Communication (changes subject rather than answer the question)
- Assertion (does not define, and states he does not wish to use)
- Nonresponsive to group role-play activity
- Sitting with head down and eyes closed during group
- Self-expression (verbal and nonverbal)

These behaviors limit his appropriate social participation and his likelihood of leaving the institution.

Progress/Rehab Potential:
- Neat appearance
- Attended group and was on time
- Remained for duration of group

A: *Poor ability to define assertive behavior and the statement that he prefers manipulation and aggression as relational skills limit Mr. S's ability to resolve conflicts and relate to others effectively, thus limiting his ability to function ① in a community setting. Lack of participation in group activity limits ability to explore alternate ways of communicating with others. Ability to manage time, willingness to remain in group until the end, and good dressing/grooming skills indicate good potential to meet stated goal of moving to next level of least restrictive environment.*

P: *Client to participate in all regularly scheduled psychosocial skills groups for 1 month, in addition to weekly 1:1 session on unit to offer opportunities to relate effectively. Focus will be on increasing participation in group activities in order to improve effective communication skills with others.*

WORKSHEET 11-12: REVISING THE "ALMOST" NOTE

✦ The "S" would be better if the therapist had asked pertinent questions, such as what the client's pain levels were.

✦ The OT is mixing her "O" data and her "A" data.

✦ There is nothing in the "O" to show that skilled OT is being provided. The list of observations of assist levels fails to provide the richness of skill used in treatment. The therapist erroneously puts some of that information in the "A" section, rather than assessing her data. In the "A" she tells us:

Client ① in dressing EOB, but is min Ⓐ in dressing when standing with a walker. Ⓛ UE AROM is WFL but Ⓡ UE has deficits noted in shoulder flexion. Client needs SBA in bed mobility when rolling to unaffected side and min Ⓐ in sit → stand 2° ↓ UE strength. Client needs SBA for transfer to unaffected side in pivot transfer bed → w/c and min Ⓐ w/c → toilet.

Even if this information were moved into the "O," there is nothing to tell us what part of the task the assistance was for.

✦ The therapist used a nonstandard abbreviation of "VCs." She means verbal cues, but since VC is a standard health term meaning *vital capacity*, it is inappropriate in its usage here.

✦ The coordination deficits mentioned in the "A" section come out of the blue. There is no mention of coordination in the opening statement (*to work on dressing and functional mobility during ADLs*), nor is it mentioned anywhere else in the "O." Thus, the statement that coordination deficits are one of the problems noted and the statement that the client would benefit from coordination exercises are unsubstantiated. Remember not to introduce any new information in the "A" section of your note.

✦ There is no real assessment of the meaning of the data found in the "S" and the "O." There is a short list of problem areas, but no assessment of their impact on the ability to engage in meaningful occupation, and no assessment of the rehab potential shown by the client's willingness to "*do whatever it takes to get out of the hospital.*"

✦ The best thing for this therapist to do is to rewrite the "O" section, providing a more comprehensive picture of the treatment session. Then she needs to assess her data based on her observations. There needs to be an indication of how the observed data impact the occupational performance of the client, before the statements about what the client would benefit from.

✦ Depending on the assessment she makes, the plan to work on balance may be appropriate, but it is likely to be only one of the things to be addressed.

CHAPTER 12

WORKSHEET 12-1: CHOOSING INTERVENTION STRATEGIES

STG	Interventions
Client will be ① in managing financial affairs within 3 weeks.	1. *Teach basic math skills (add, subtract, multiply, divide).* 2. *Role play to make change correctly.* 3. *Set-up task for writing checks to pay fabricated bills.* 4. *Teach comparison shopping using a catalog.* 5. *Set-up task of writing out a budget.* 6. *Set-up task of balancing checkbook.* 7. *Set-up experience for deciding whether a given amount of money will be enough for living expenses once a set of fabricated bills has been paid.*

WORKSHEET 12-2: WRITING THE ASSESSMENT AND INTERVENTION PLAN: THE CASE OF GEORGIA S

A: ↓ *activity tolerance and standing balance, weakness in* Ⓑ *shoulder flex/abd, and* ↓ *problem-solving skills result in* ↓ *safety &* Ⓘ *in dressing & grooming.* ↓ *standing balance impairs safe and* Ⓘ *functional mobility during ADLs. Weak grasp and pinch of* Ⓡ *hand and* ↓ *coordination impairs fine motor ADL tasks including donning sock and brushing teeth. Rehab potential is good for returning home with caregiver assistance. Client would benefit from continued OT to increase activity tolerance, dynamic standing balance, and safety for ADL tasks.*

P: *Pt. to be seen b.i.d for 45-minute sessions for 3 weeks to* ↑ Ⓘ *in self-care activities. Client will be instructed in adaptive equipment/techniques. Interventions will also focus on* ↑ *activity tolerance, standing balance, and* Ⓘ *in functional mobility for ADLs, and* ↑ Ⓡ *hand strength in order to complete dressing and toileting* Ⓘ.

Strengths: Ⓘ *in self-care prior to CVA; able to ambulate* c̄ *walker; intact sensation except* Ⓡ *hand stereognosis; all UE AROM WNL or WFL*

Functional Problem Statement #1: *Impaired problem solving,* ↓ *coordination,* ↓ *stereognosis, and* ↓ *standing balance impair ability to perform self-care tasks* Ⓘ.

Long-Term Goal #1: *Client will complete all dressing and grooming tasks with modified* Ⓘ *using walker for tasks set-up by anticipated discharge on 7/03/11.*

STGs (Objectives)	Interventions
STG #1: *Client will don/doff gown and robe with min* Ⓐ *and verbal cues by 6/17/11.*	1. *Instruct client in upper body dressing techniques and have client demonstrate over-the-head and button-up methods, first in sitting, then progress to standing.* 2. *Provide tactile cues to use alternative techniques.* 3. *Have client problem solve next step of dressing or grooming tasks in sequence using visual aid and then verbal cues as needed. Ask client what to do next or why this is not working now.* 4. *Engage client in reaching activities that provide a graded challenge to balance.* 5. *Engage client in activities that* ↑ *AROM and fine motor tasks such as buttoning and zipping that are graded for level of difficulty in coordination.*
STG #2: *By 6/24/11, client will complete grooming tasks standing at sink for at least 10 minutes with CGA for balance and one 30-sec rest break.*	1. *Educate client on identifying signs of fatigue. Plan rest breaks as needed to* ↓ *fatigue.* 2. *Perform tabletop activities including self-care tasks with time increasing as tolerated.* 3. *Perform deep breathing exercises and instruct in energy conservation techniques.* 4. *Instruct client in theraputty exercises to be performed in room in between OT sessions to increase grip and pinch strength.*

Functional Problem Statement #2: *Fatigue during ADLs and* ↓ *dynamic balance during toileting raise safety concern for being home alone during the day.*

Long-Term Goal #2: *By discharge on 7/03/11, client will perform toileting with modified independence using a walker and bedside commode.*

STGs (Objectives)	Interventions
STG #1: *In 1 week, client will transfer safely ↔ 3-in-1 commode for toileting with min Ⓐ to manage clothing and no more than 2 verbal cues.*	1. *Instruct client in safe transfer techniques; reinforce compliance when transferring ↔ bed, armchairs, commode, and mat for therapeutic activities, strengthening exercises, toileting, or dressing activities.* 2. *Provide Ⓡ UE strengthening and AROM through reaching and weightbearing activities such as reaching at sink for grooming and dressing items in graded challenging positions, pushing up from armchair and bedside commode, and table top activities of interest that require alternating support on one arm while actively reaching with the other.*
STG #2: *In 2 weeks, client will transfer safely ↔ 3-in-1 commode for toileting with SBA to manage clothing and no more than 1 verbal cue.*	1. *Continue with transfer education and practice.* 2. *Interview client and daughter regarding home environment; explore and discuss equipment use & placement in home; discuss support services needed if discharge to home is warranted.* 3. *Schedule a home visit for assessment of client's ability to manage in home environment.*

Discharge Plan: *To home if environmental adaptations and support of caregiver and/or services are available. If client is not Ⓘ in self-care activities by 7/03/11, the recommendation would be to discharge to a skilled nursing facility for 2-3 weeks until self-care goals are met.*

Signature: *Shannon M, OTR/L*

WORKSHEET 12-3: PLANNING INTERVENTIONS USING GROUPS—HEATHER'S SUICIDE ATTEMPT

Problem #1: Exacerbation of depressive symptoms resulting in a suicide attempt.
LTG #1: By anticipated discharge in 4 days, Heather will demonstrate improved self-esteem by verbally identifying strengths, caring for her appearance, making eye contact when interacting with others, and developing a plan for coping with suicidal thoughts.

Interventions	
Goals Group	1. *Listen attentively to Heather when she shares her goal.* 2. *Offer eye contact and offer Heather the opportunity to make eye contact in return before cueing her.* 3. *Help Heather identify the relationship between her values and her daily goals (i.e., a goal to wash her hair if related to valuing a neat and clean appearance).* 4. *Help Heather break down larger goals (such as "be happy") into smaller accomplishable and measurable increments.* 5. *Show respect for Heather's choices.* 6. *Provide feedback on Heather's successes in meeting her daily goals.* 7. *Facilitate goal choices that show increased self-esteem.* 8. *Compliment Heather on her appearance when any part of her appearance shows more attention to her self-care.* 9. *Facilitate goal choices that involve taking care of herself.*

Stress Management Group	1. *Welcome Heather by greeting her warmly, sitting by her, or smiling.*
	2. *Offer opportunities to identify strengths through visualization and imagery.*
	3. *Help Heather identify stresses that led her to recent suicide attempt.*
	4. *Help Heather identify stresses that occur frequently.*
	5. *Help Heather identify physical and behavioral changes that occur when she experiences stress.*
	6. *Help Heather identify both successful and unsuccessful stress relief strategies that she has used in the past.*
	7. *Brainstorm ways of handling stressful situations that seem overwhelming before those situations become life-threatening.*
	8. *Use positive affirmations.*
	9. *Provide practice for a variety of stress management strategies.*
	10. *Develop a plan for managing stress when feeling overwhelmed.*
IADL Group	1. *Identify strengths about each person through group discussion, art activities (draw your best quality, personality collage, etc.), and games.*
	2. *Use a peer feedback activity that gives group members opportunities to identify and recognize each other's strengths.*
	3. *Offer quick success projects, such as putting together jewelry, making bookmarks, or completing small kits.*
	4. *Ask Heather for her ideas about how best to use the group time.*
	5. *Note aspects of Heather's work that are executed with competence.*
	6. *In a group that is all women, learn to apply make-up or style hair.*

Problem #2: Stress related to recent role changes result in Heather's inability to concentrate and make decisions for her daily life.

LTG #2: Heather will apply a decision-making strategy to her two most important current life decisions by discharge in 4 days.

Interventions	
Goals Group	1. *Identify a small accomplishment goal for the day.*
	2. *Help Heather identify what is realistic to accomplish in 1 day.*
	3. *Help Heather make her goal measurable.*
	4. *Write that goal on a card for Heather to carry with her throughout the day.*
	5. *Make a verbal contract with Heather to accomplish her goal.*
	6. *Teach the relationship between setting daily goals and making larger life decisions.*
	7. *Follow-up daily on Heather's goal for the day.*
	8. *Encourage Heather to make goals related to major life stressors.*
Stress Management Group	1. *Help Heather identify triggers in her environment that cause a stress reaction.*
	2. *Help Heather identify negative thoughts that increase her stress level. Instruct Heather on how to replace them with more positive and realistic thoughts.*
	3. *Help Heather bring her thoughts to the present moment and to come back into the present moment when she drifts into the past and future.*
	4. *Use movement, such as stretching or progressive relaxation, to help Heather focus on the task at hand.*

IADL Group	1. *Ask Heather what strategies she uses to focus her mind.*
	2. *Plan group topics around Heather's current issues, such as: ways of getting to sleep, overcoming loneliness, and feeling worthwhile.*
	3. *Use a cognitively stimulating activity to help Heather focus.*
	4. *Instruct Heather on a problem-solving strategy and practice applying it to sample problems.*
	5. *Brainstorm strategies for making good decisions and rank these in effectiveness.*
	6. *Ask Heather to identify one major decision needing to be made, and list pros/cons of each possible course of action.*
	7. *Role play a decision-making situation.*
	8. *Use games that require decision making.*
	9. *Adapt tasks so that Heather will be able to concentrate on a task long enough to complete it.*

Problem #3: Inability to manage anger constructively resulting in behaviors that damage self, relationships, and property.

LTG #3: By anticipated discharge in 4 days, Heather independently will identify potential anger triggers, her physical reactions to being angry, and develop a plan to prevent escalation and destructive behaviors.

Interventions	
Goals Group	1. *Use active listening to help Heather identify feelings related to her goals.*
	2. *Ask Heather about daily incidents involving anger and encourage goals for useful solutions if incidents arise.*
Stress Management Group	1. *Use stress management techniques that focus on body sensations.*
	2. *Teach Heather to focus on the breath to bring her to the present moment, to relax, and to enhance sleep.*
	3. *Invite Heather to identify and express feelings that arise during the exercises.*
	4. *Use sounds and recordings that activate the parasympathetic nervous system.*
	5. *Identify strategies for restful sleep and encourage her to practice these at night.*
IADL Group	1. *Teach anger management strategies.*
	2. *Help Heather identify potential anger-provoking situations.*
	3. *Help Heather identify early physical signs of escalating anger.*
	4. *Help Heather develop a plan for what to do when she notices her anger beginning to escalate.*
	5. *Help Heather identify safe outlets for anger to prevent it from escalating.*
	6. *Instruct Heather on constructive ways to communicate her anger to others.*
	7. *Help Heather identify feelings that arise during the group.*
	8. *Use sounds and language to elicit feelings.*
	9. *Use art activities to explore and express feelings.*
	10. *Identify stressors that trigger anger through group discussion, adapted games, or art.*
	11. *Role play situations around anger and frustration.*
	12. *Identify social supports (friends, family, support groups, crisis lines) to use when angry.*
	13. *Teach and role play problem solving.*
	14. *Coach Heather as she practices managing anger with phone calls and visitors.*
	15. *Teach the use of an "anger continuum" to recognize varying degrees and experiences of anger.*

Index

Wait...There's More!

SLACK Incorporated's Health Care Books and Journals offers a wide selection of books in the field of Occupational Therapy. We are dedicated to providing important works that educate, inform and improve the knowledge of our customers. Don't miss out on our other informative titles that will enhance your collection.

Quick Reference Dictionary for Occupational Therapy, Fifth Edition
Karen Jacobs EdD, OTR/L, CPE, FAOTA;
Laela Jacobs, OTR

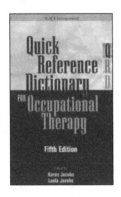

632 pp., Soft Cover, 2009, ISBN 13 978-1-55642-865-4, Order# 38654, **$43.95**

This handy dictionary provides a quick reference to words, their definitions, and important resources that are used in daily practice and academic training. Its convenient size makes it easy to use whether you're in the clinic or at school.

Occupational Therapy Interventions:
Function and Occupations
Catherine Meriano, JD, MHS, OTR/L;
Donna Latella, EdD, OTR/L

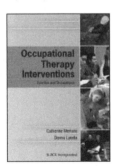

560 pp., Soft Cover, 2008, ISBN 13 978-1-55642-732-9, Order# 47328, **$50.95**

Throughout this text, Catherine Meriano and Donna Latella provide a hands-on approach to the physical dysfunction intervention process while covering all performance areas in the *Occupational Therapy Practice Framework*.

Documentation Manual for Writing SOAP Notes in Occupational Therapy, Third Edition
Crystal Gateley, MA, OTR/L; Sherry Borcherding, MA, OTR/L
264 pp., Soft Cover, 2012, ISBN 13 978-1-55642-971-2, Order# 39712, **$49.95**

Group Dynamics in Occupational Therapy:
The Theoretical Basis and Practice Application of Group Intervention, Fourth Edition
Marilyn B. Cole, MS, OTR/L, FAOTA
435 pp., Soft Cover, 2011, ISBN 13 978-1-55642-011-5, Order# 30115, **$59.95**

Occupational Therapy: Performance, Participation, and Well-Being, Third Edition
Charles H. Christiansen, EdD, OTR, OT(C), FAOTA;
Carolyn M. Baum, PhD, OTR/L, FAOTA; Julie Bass Haugen, PhD, OTR/L, FAOTA; Julie D. Bass, PhD, OTR/L, FAOTA
680 pp., Hard Cover, 2005, ISBN 13 978-1-55642-530-1, Order# 35309, **$77.95**

Vision, Perception, and Cognition:
A Manual for the Evaluation and Treatment of the Adult With Acquired Brain Injury, Fourth Edition
Barbara Zoltan, MA, OTR/L
368 pp., Hard Cover, 2007, ISBN 13 978-1-55642-738-1, Order# 37387, **$52.95**

Crafts and Creative Media in Therapy, Third Edition
Carol Tubbs, MA, OTR/L;
Margaret Drake, PhD, OTR/L, ATR-BC, LPAT, FAOTA
304 pp., Soft Cover, 2007, ISBN 13 978-1-55642-756-5, Order# 37565, **$51.95**

Please visit **www.slackbooks.com** to order any of the above titles!
24 Hours a Day...7 Days a Week!

WRITING PROBLEM STATEMENTS

For ease of writing, you can use the following formula to write a functional problem statement:

Client requires _____ in _____ due to _____.
                    assist level   performing what occupational task   contributing factor

+ *Child requires mod (A) to hold scissors to complete art activities in school due to high tone in (R) UE.*
+ *Veteran requires min (A) in completing toilet transfer due to trunk instability resulting from (R) CVA.*
+ *Consumer requires maximal verbal cues to complete 3-step lunch preparation due to decreased sequencing and problem-solving skills.*

If a client is unable to perform an activity independently, the assist level will be specified. However, sometimes the activity is one that the client either **can** or **cannot** do, with no assist levels in question. In that case, you can use the following format:

Client unable to _____ due to _____.
                     engage in what occupational task   what contributing factor

+ *Consumer is unable to sustain employment more than 2 weeks due to absence of stress management skills.*
+ *Client is unable to grasp a writing instrument for more than 3 minutes due to pain level of >5/10 with finger flexion of (R) hand.*
+ *Child is unable to do jumping jacks to participate in gym class due to motor planning deficits.*

It is not mandatory that the formats above be used. These are useful ways of wording functional problem statements, but there are others. Sometimes a slightly different format is more useful:

_____ results in _____.
      Contributing factor   what occupational deficit

+ *Three steps leading to front door limit client's independence in entering house.*
+ *Inability to perform simple math calculations results in need for caregiver assistance in IADL tasks such as balancing checkbook.*
+ *Pain level >6 at end range shoulder flexion limits ability to don shirt overhead.*
+ *Aggressive behavior results in limited opportunities for social participation and repeated involvement with the juvenile justice system.*

Goal Writing: The COAST Method

- ✦ C–Client   Client will perform
- ✦ O–Occupation   What occupation?
- ✦ A–Assist Level   With what level of assistance/independence?
- ✦ S–Specific Condition   Under what conditions?
- ✦ T–Timeline   By when?

Example:
- ✦ C: *Client will perform*
- ✦ O: *bed making activity*
- ✦ A: *with min verbal cues*
- ✦ S: *while adhering to post-surgical back precautions*
- ✦ T: *by 12/12/11.*

The "A" and "S" together make your goal statement **measurable** and allow you to show your client's progress. In some cases, it is acceptable to omit either the "A" or the "S," **but never both**.

As long as all the required elements are present, it does not matter with which element you begin your sentence.

- ✦ *Client will prepare a 3-step meal in rehab kitchen with modified independence from wheelchair level within 2 weeks.*
- ✦ *Within 3 treatment sessions, Mr. S will complete toileting using raised toilet seat with min Ⓐ for balance during clothing adjustment.*
- ✦ *Client will analyze bill statement and write check for correct amount 3 of 4 attempts with min verbal cues by 8/19/11.*
- ✦ *By the end of the school year, child will copy 10 math problems from whiteboard to paper with <2 errors and no verbal cues, 80% of attempts.*
- ✦ *Client will transfer 10# boxes from floor to shelf during simulated work tasks, demonstrating proper body mechanics without verbal cues by 10/17/11.*
- ✦ *Child will catch tennis ball in Ⓑ hands 8 of 10 attempts when tossed from 10 feet within 3 weeks.*
- ✦ *Deondré will make at least 2 verbal contributions to group discussions with min verbal prompts 5/5 days within 2 weeks.*
- ✦ *Client independently will identify at least 3 leisure activities that are not associated with drinking by 9/08/11.*
- ✦ *Client will demonstrate ability to change infant's diaper using adaptive one-handed methods with 2 or fewer verbal cues within 2 weeks.*

A QUICK CHECKLIST FOR EVALUATING YOUR NOTE

Use the following summary chart as a quick-reference guide to be sure that your note contains all of the essential elements.

	S:
☐	Use something significant that the client says about his or her treatment or condition.
	O:
☐	Begin with a statement about the length, setting, and purpose of the treatment session, using wording that indicates active participation by the client.
☐	Follow the opening statement with a summary of what you have observed, either chronologically or using categories.
☐	Be professional, concise, and specific.
☐	Focus on occupation.
☐	Focus on the client's response to the treatment provided, rather than on what the therapist did.
☐	Write from the client's point of view, leaving yourself out.
☐	Be specific about assist levels.
☐	Avoid making a list of actions and assist levels.
☐	De-emphasize the treatment media.
☐	Make certain that it is clear that you were not just a passive observer in the session.
☐	Avoid judging the client.
☐	Use only standard abbreviations.
	A:
☐	Go sentence by sentence through the information presented in the "S" and the "O," asking yourself what it means for the client's ability to engage in meaningful occupation. Note what **problems**, **progress**, and **potential** for rehabilitation you see.
☐	Remember the formula that puts the contributing factor as the subject of your sentence:
	<table><tr><td>Contributing Factor</td><td>Impact</td><td>Ability to Engage in Occupation</td></tr></table>
☐	End the "A" with "*Client would benefit from....*," justifying continued skilled OT and setting up the plan.
☐	Be sure that the time lines and activities you are putting in your plan match the skilled OT you say your client needs.
	P:
☐	Specify the frequency and duration of future OT sessions (e.g., 2x/wk for 4 wks).
☐	Describe the purpose of future OT sessions.
☐	Include a brief description of the intervention strategies that will address the client's goals.

If you have read the text carefully, you will know what each item means. For a more complete explanation, refer to the chapter that provides information in detail.

S:

+ Use something significant that the client says about his or her treatment or condition. If there is nothing significant, ask yourself whether you are using your interview skills effectively to elicit the information about the client's perspective.

O:

+ Begin with a statement about the length, setting, and purpose of the treatment session, using wording that indicates active participation by the client.

    Client participated in 45-minute OT session in rehab kitchen for meal preparation activity.

+ Focus on the client's response, rather than on what you did.

    Client able to don socks using sock-aid after demonstration.

+ Write from the client's point of view, leaving yourself out.

    Client repositioned rather than *Therapist repositioned client.*

+ Be specific about assist levels.

    Client required min Ⓐ for hand placement during pivot transfer to toilet.

+ De-emphasize the treatment media.

    Client worked on tripod pinch using pegs in order to grasp objects needed for ADLs.

+ Make certain that it is clear that you were not just a passive observer in the session. Don't just make a list of all the assist levels and think that is enough.

+ Avoid judging the client. For example, say he "*...didn't complete the activity.*" Don't add "*...because he was stubborn.*"

A:

+ Go sentence by sentence through the information presented in the "S" and the "O," asking yourself what it means for the client's ability to engage in meaningful occupation. Note what **problems**, **progress**, and **potential** for rehabilitation you see.

+ Remember the formula that puts the contributing factor as the subject of your sentence:

Contributing Factor	Impact	Ability to Engage in Occupation

Deficits in UE AROM & strength limit client's ability to complete basic self-care tasks.

+ End the "A" with "*Client would benefit from....,*" justifying continued skilled OT and setting up the plan.

    Client would benefit from skilled instruction in energy conservation techniques, continued strengthening of UE, and compensatory techniques for performing IADLs one-handed.

P:

+ Specify frequency, duration, and purpose of future sessions, and give a brief description of planned interventions.

    Infant will be seen 2x/wk. for 2 months to address feeding skills. Treatment to include oral desensitization and caregiver training in use of adaptive bottles.